CW01263168

A GUIDE FOR

International Nursing Students

IN

Australia and New Zealand

A GUIDE FOR International Nursing Students IN Australia and New Zealand

M Bernadette Hally

CHURCHILL LIVINGSTONE
ELSEVIER

Sydney Edinburgh London New York Philadelphia St Louis Toronto

ELSEVIER

Churchill Livingstone
is an imprint of Elsevier

Elsevier Australia. ACN 001 002 357
(a division of Reed International Books Australia Pty Ltd)
Tower 1, 475 Victoria Avenue, Chatswood, NSW 2067

National Library of Australia Cataloguing-in-Publication Data

---

Hally, M. Bernadette.

A guide for international nursing students in Australia and New Zealand/M Bernadette Hally.

ISBN: 978 0 7295 3879 4 (pbk.)

Includes bibliographical references and index.

Communication in nursing. Nursing—Australia.
Nurses, Foreign—Australia.
Nursing—New Zealand.
Nurses, Foreign—New Zealand.

610.73069

Publisher: Luisa Cecotti
Developmental Editor: Sabrina Chew
Publishing Services Manager: Helena Klijn
Editorial Coordinator: Eleanor Cant
Edited by Ruth Matheson
Proofread by Brenda Hamilton
Cover & internal design by Toni Darben
Index by Deirdre Ward
Typeset by Pindar NZ, Auckland, New Zealand
Printed by Ligare

This book is dedicated to Joe and Xavier:
the loves and light of my life.

CONTENTS

CONTENTS

Foreword

This book is invaluable in preparing international nurses and international nursing students to practise in Australia and New Zealand. There has been a need for such a book for a long time—to assist the growing numbers of nurses and prospective nurses who are required to deal with the intricacies of practising as a registered nurse in Australia and New Zealand. This is often very different from nursing in other countries.

This high-quality book clearly explains the role of the nurse, the health systems in Australia and New Zealand, and, most importantly, the language used by nurses when they communicate with each other, their patients and doctors. This jargon or informal language is unique, and not taught in the English language courses that international nurses or students undertake.

The book is supported with a CD, which allows the reader to listen to words or expressions and to the English as it is spoken by the nurse. This CD is an excellent resource that supports the text in the book. Each chapter features learning objectives, key terms, reflective questions, chapter highlights and self-test questions that are easy to follow and further assist the reader with their self-learning by encouraging readers to review their understanding of the content.

There are considerable benefits for the overseas registered nurse and/or student in reading this book prior to undertaking clinical practice in Australia or New Zealand. This book draws on the vast experience of the author in working with and teaching international nursing students. As the Head of a large nursing school, with hundreds of international nursing students, I have often seen the problems and issues faced by students when they enter the clinical areas. I will be recommending this excellent textbook to all international students in my School—to be read at the beginning of their studies.

Associate Professor Michelle Campbell
Head, School of Nursing and Midwifery (Victoria)
Australian Catholic University

Preface to the student

This text has been written with the intention of developing a resource that brings together the essential content for the international nurse and nursing student, and creating a comprehensive 'must have' guide for the reader. The learning activities throughout the text and on the CD are intended to provide the reader with the opportunity to develop knowledge and skills for study and nursing practice.

The text is divided into seven parts. Parts 1–6 each have a number of chapters that address important aspects of nursing in Australia and New Zealand. Part 7 contains learning activities for use with the CD Part 1—Audio, 'Nursing conversations' (A4–A14) and 'Nursing handovers' (A15–A16). Each chapter can be used as a discrete learning module, and includes questions for reflection, self-test questions and suggestions for learning.

The CD is divided into three parts:

- Part 1 is the **audio** component. You can hear the pronunciation of colloquialisms, phrasal verbs and acronyms (A1–A3), and you can listen to 'Nursing conversations' (A4–A14) and 'Nursing handovers' (A15–A16).
- Part 2 contains the **transcripts** for the audio component, so that you can practise the pronunciation of expressions and terminology, improve your listening skills and develop your vocabulary.
- Part 3 contains **reader resources**, including the 'Article summary sheet' (R1) and the 'Language list' (R2) that you will use when completing the 'Self-test questions' at the end of most chapters, along with checklists, sample documents, templates, self-directed learning packages and a set of sample hospital documents. These resources are designed to assist your study and clinical practice.

Throughout the text, you will be advised when to listen to the CD.

It is hoped that this text will be a valuable resource for all international nurses and nursing students—and their teachers—in Australia and New Zealand.

Recommended resources to support your learning

International students who are completing full undergraduate programs will be referred to many other resources in their studies. For those who are completing specialised programs, or who are already working, the following table contains some key resources (which are cited in the text or listed as 'Recommended reading' at the end of chapters) for supporting your learning.

RECOMMENDED RESOURCES

Content	Reference
Fundamentals/foundations of nursing	Crisp J, Taylor C (eds) 2009 Potter & Perry's fundamentals of nursing, 3rd edn. Elsevier, Sydney
Medical-surgical nursing	Brown D, Edwards H (eds) 2008 Lewis's medical-surgical nursing: assessment and management of clinical problems, 2nd edn. Elsevier, Sydney
Mental health nursing	Elder R, Evans K, Nizette D (eds) 2008 Psychiatric and mental health nursing, 2nd edn. Elsevier, Sydney Fortinash KM, Holoday Worret PA 2007 Psychiatric mental health nursing, 4th edn. Elsevier, St Louis
Clinical nursing skills	Perry AG, Potter PA 2005 Clinical nursing skills and techniques, 6th edn. Elsevier, St Louis Tollefson J 2004 Clinical psychomotor skills: assessment tools for nursing students, 2nd edn. Social Science Press, Tuggerah
Drug calculations	Gatford JD, Phillips N 2006 Nursing calculations, 7th edn. Elsevier, Edinburgh
Clinical placement	Levett-Jones T, Bourgeois S 2007 The clinical placement: an essential guide for nursing students. Elsevier, Sydney
Medical-nursing dictionary	Harris P, Nagy S, Vardaxis N (eds) 2005 Mosby's medical, nursing and allied health dictionary: (Australia/New Zealand edition). Elsevier, Sydney
Australia: codes and competencies for nurses (see Ch 5 for complete citations and sources)	Code of Ethics for Nurses in Australia, June 2002
	Code of Professional Conduct for Nurses in Australia, January 2003
	National Competency Standards for the Registered Nurse, 4th edn, January 2006
	National Competency Standards for the Enrolled Nurse, October 2002
New Zealand: codes, guidelines and competencies for nurses (see Ch 5 for complete citations and sources)	Code of Conduct for Nurses, March 2008
	Guidelines for Cultural Safety, the Treaty of Waitangi and Māori Health in Nursing Education and Practice, March 2005
	Competencies for Registered Nurses, December 2007
	Competencies for Nurse Assistants and Enrolled Nurses, December 2007

A **chapter outline** introduces each chapter to give you an overview of the chapter's contents.

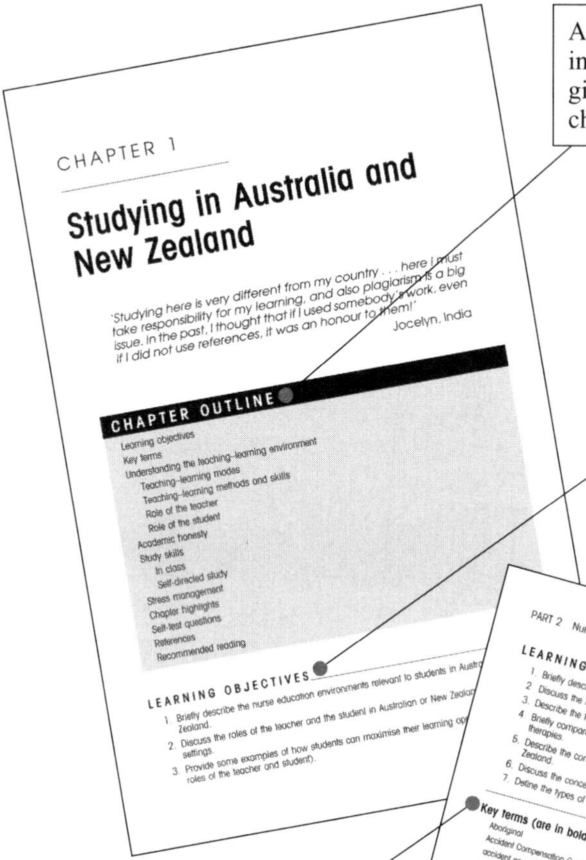

CHAPTER 1

Studying in Australia and New Zealand

'Studying here is very different from my country . . . here I must take responsibility for my learning, and also plagiarism is a big issue. In the past, I thought that if I used somebody's work, even if I did not use references, it was an honour to them!'
Jocelyn, India

CHAPTER OUTLINE

Learning objectives
Key terms
Understanding the teaching–learning environment
Teaching–learning modes
Teaching–learning methods and skills
Role of the teacher
Role of the student
Academic honesty
Study skills
In class
Self-directed study
Stress management
Chapter highlights
Self-test questions
References
Recommended reading

LEARNING OBJECTIVES

1. Briefly describe the nurse education environments relevant to students in Austra[lia]
2. Discuss the roles of the teacher and the student in Australian or New Zealan[d] settings.
3. Provide some examples of how students can maximise their learning op[portunities] roles of the teacher and student).

Learning objectives at the beginning of each chapter help you to focus on the key information that follows and can be used as self-test questions when revising the topic.

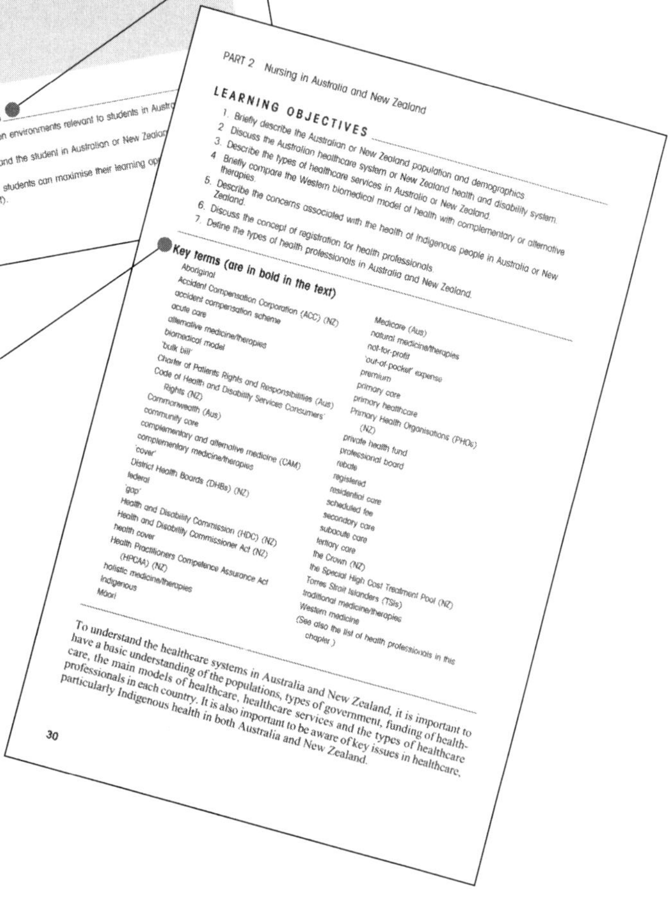

PART 2 Nursing in Australia and New Zealand

LEARNING OBJECTIVES

1. Briefly describe the Australian or New Zealand population and demographics.
2. Discuss the Australian healthcare system or New Zealand health and disability system.
3. Describe the types of healthcare services in Australia or New Zealand.
4. Briefly compare the Western biomedical model of health with complementary or alternative therapies.
5. Describe the concerns associated with the health of Indigenous people in Australia or New Zealand.
6. Discuss the concept of registration for health professionals.
7. Define the types of health professionals in Australia and New Zealand.

Key terms (are in bold in the text)

Aboriginal
Accident Compensation Corporation (ACC) (NZ)
accident compensation scheme
acute care
alternative medicine/therapies
biomedical model
'bulk bill'
Charter of Patients Rights and Responsibilities (Aus)
Code of Health and Disability Services Consumers' Rights (NZ)
Commonwealth (Aus)
community care
complementary and alternative medicine (CAM)
complementary medicine/therapies
'cover'
District Health Boards (DHBs) (NZ)
federal
'gap'
Health and Disability Commission (HDC) (NZ)
Health and Disability Commissioner Act (NZ)
health cover
Health Practitioners Competence Assurance Act (HPCAA) (NZ)
holistic medicine/therapies
Indigenous
Māori
Medicare (Aus)
natural medicine/therapies
not-for-profit
'out-of-pocket' expense
premium
primary care
primary healthcare
Primary Health Organisations (PHOs) (NZ)
private health fund
professional board
rebate
registered
residential care
scheduled fee
secondary care
subacute care
tertiary care
the Crown (NZ)
the Special High Cost Treatment Pool (NZ)
Torres Strait Islanders (TSIs)
traditional medicine/therapies
Western medicine
(See also the list of health professionals in this chapter.)

To understand the healthcare systems in Australia and New Zealand, it is important to have a basic understanding of the populations, types of government, funding of healthcare, the main models of healthcare, healthcare services and the types of healthcare professionals in each country. It is also important to be aware of key issues in healthcare, particularly Indigenous health in both Australia and New Zealand.

30

Key terms are listed at the beginning of each chapter to assist your vocabulary development. The acronyms for key terms are listed in brackets following the term. If relevant only in Australia, 'Aus' is noted beside the term; if relevant only in New Zealand, 'NZ' is noted beside the term. Each key term is also highlighted in **bold** where it is discussed in the chapter.

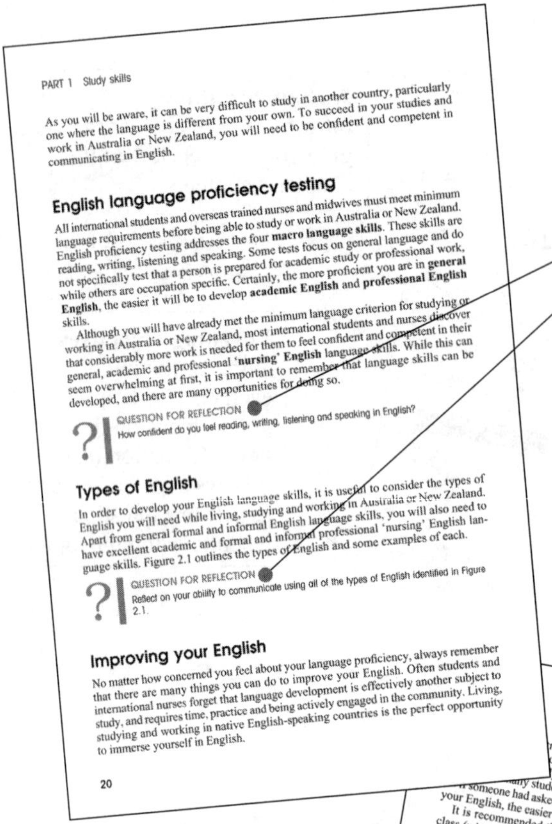

PART 1 Study skills

As you will be aware, it can be very difficult to study in another country, particularly one where the language is different from your own. To succeed in your studies and work in Australia or New Zealand, you will need to be confident and competent in communicating in English.

English language proficiency testing

All international students and overseas trained nurses and midwives must meet minimum language requirements before being able to study or work in Australia or New Zealand. English proficiency testing addresses the four **macro language skills**. These skills are reading, writing, listening and speaking. Some tests focus on general language and do not specifically test that a person is prepared for academic study or professional work, while others are occupation specific. Certainly, the more proficient you are in **general English**, the easier it will be to develop **academic English** and **professional English** skills.

Although you will have already met the minimum language criterion for studying or working in Australia or New Zealand, most international students and nurses discover that considerably more work is needed for them to feel confident and competent in their general, academic and professional '**nursing**' **English** language skills. While this can seem overwhelming at first, it is important to remember that language skills can be developed, and there are many opportunities for doing so.

QUESTION FOR REFLECTION

How confident do you feel reading, writing, listening and speaking in English?

Types of English

In order to develop your English language skills, it is useful to consider the types of English you will need while living, studying and working in Australia or New Zealand. Apart from general formal and informal English language skills, you will also need to have excellent academic and formal and informal professional 'nursing' English language skills. Figure 2.1 outlines the types of English and some examples of each.

QUESTION FOR REFLECTION

Reflect on your ability to communicate using all of the types of English identified in Figure 2.1.

Improving your English

No matter how concerned you feel about your language proficiency, always remember that there are many things you can do to improve your English. Often students and international nurses forget that language development is effectively another subject to study, and requires time, practice and being actively engaged in the community. Living, studying and working in native English-speaking countries is the perfect opportunity to immerse yourself in English.

20

Questions for reflection help you to think about important ideas and issues.

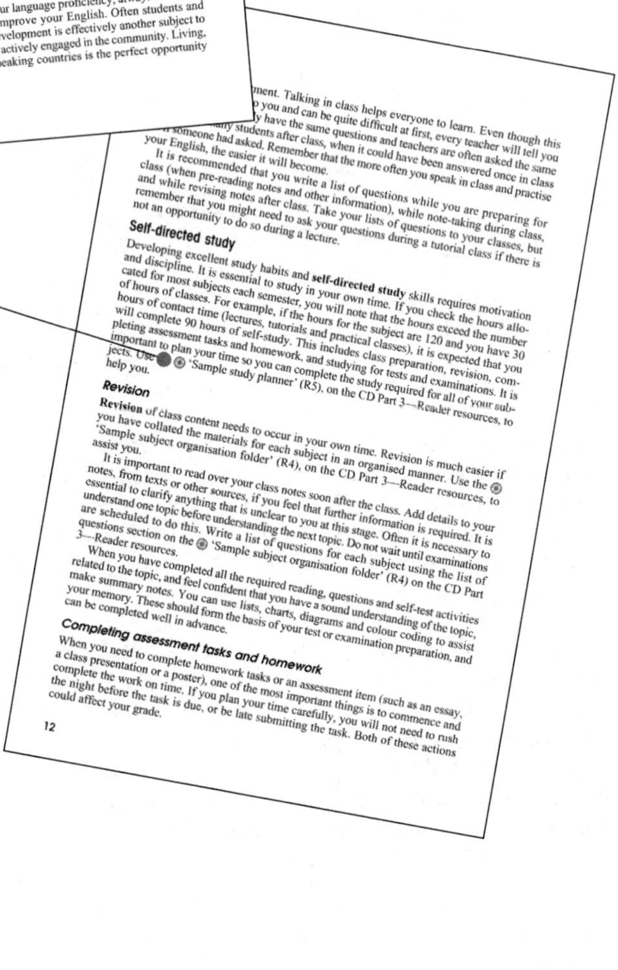

...ment. Talking in class helps everyone to learn. Even though this ...o you and can be quite difficult at first, every teacher will tell you ...y have the same questions and teachers are often asked the same ...any students after class, when it could have been answered once in class ...someone had asked. Remember that the more often you speak in class and practise your English, the easier it will become.

It is recommended that you write a list of questions while you are preparing for class (when pre-reading notes and other information), while note-taking during class, and while revising notes after class. Take your lists of questions to your classes, but remember that you might need to ask your questions during a tutorial class if there is not an opportunity to do so during a lecture.

Self-directed study

Developing excellent study habits and **self-directed study** skills requires motivation and discipline. It is essential to study in your own time. If you check the hours allocated for most subjects each semester, you will note that the hours exceed the number of hours of classes. For example, if the hours for the subject are 120 and you have 30 hours of contact time (lectures, tutorials and practical classes), it is expected that you will complete 90 hours of self-study. This includes class preparation, revision, completing assessment tasks and homework, and studying for tests and examinations. It is important to plan your time so you can complete the study required for all of your subjects. Use the ◎ 'Sample study planner' (R5), on the CD Part 3—Reader resources, to help you.

Revision

Revision of class content needs to occur in your own time. Revision is much easier if you have collated the materials for each subject in an organised manner. Use the ◎ 'Sample subject organisation folder' (R4), on the CD Part 3—Reader resources, to assist you.

It is important to read over your class notes soon after the class. Add details to your notes, from texts or other sources, if you feel that further information is required. It is essential to clarify anything that is unclear to you at this stage. Often it is necessary to understand one topic before understanding the next topic. Do not wait until examinations are scheduled to do this. Write a list of questions for each subject using the list of questions section on the ◎ 'Sample subject organisation folder' (R4) on the CD Part 3—Reader resources.

When you have completed all the required reading, questions and self-test activities related to the topic, and feel confident that you have a sound understanding of the topic, make summary notes. You can use lists, charts, diagrams and colour coding to assist your memory. These should form the basis of your test or examination preparation, and can be completed well in advance.

Completing assessment tasks and homework

When you need to complete homework tasks or an assessment item (such as an essay, a class presentation or a poster), one of the most important things is to commence and complete the work on time. If you plan your time carefully, you will not need to rush the night before the task is due, or be late submitting the task. Both of these actions could affect your grade.

12

When you see the ◎ **CD symbol** in the text, you will be referred to the CD. The symbol tells you when you need to refer to an **audio** file on the CD (Part 1 of the CD: A1–A16), a **transcript** of one of the audio files (Part 2 of the CD: T1–T16) or one of the **reader resources** (Part 3 of the CD: R1–R13).

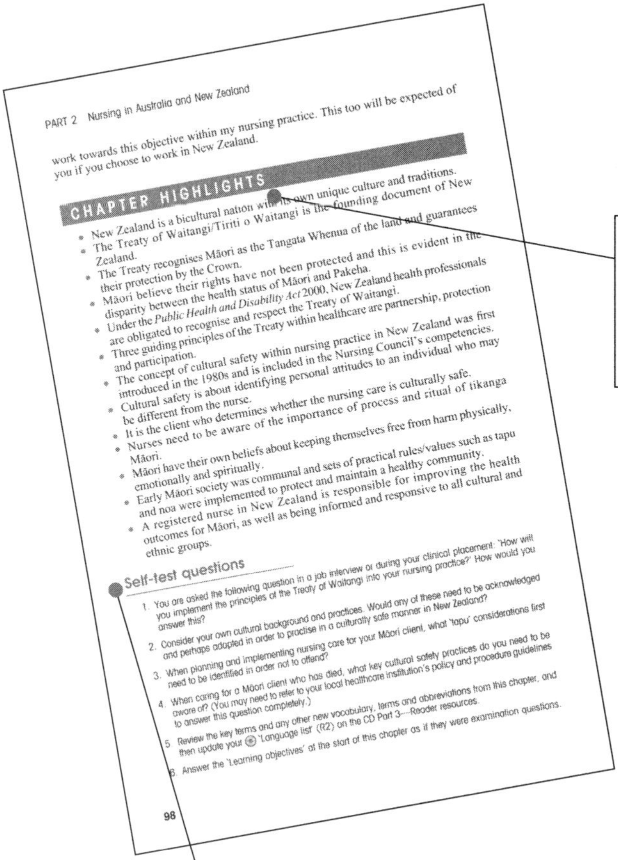

PART 2 Nursing in Australia and New Zealand

work towards this objective within my nursing practice. This too will be expected of you if you choose to work in New Zealand.

CHAPTER HIGHLIGHTS

- New Zealand is a bicultural nation with its own unique culture and traditions.
- The Treaty of Waitangi/Tiriti o Waitangi is the founding document of New Zealand.
- The Treaty recognises Māori as the Tangata Whenua of the land and guarantees their protection by the Crown.
- Māori believe their rights have not been protected and this is evident in the disparity between the health status of Māori and Pakeha.
- Under the *Public Health and Disability Act* 2000, New Zealand health professionals are obligated to recognise and respect the Treaty of Waitangi.
- Three guiding principles of the Treaty within healthcare are partnership, protection and participation.
- The concept of cultural safety within nursing practice in New Zealand was first introduced in the 1980s and is included in the Nursing Council's competencies.
- Cultural safety is about identifying personal attitudes to an individual who may be different from the nurse.
- It is the client who determines whether the nursing care is culturally safe.
- Nurses need to be aware of the importance of process and ritual of tikanga Māori.
- Māori have their own beliefs about keeping themselves free from harm physically, emotionally and spiritually.
- Early Māori society was communal and sets of practical rules/values such as tapu and noa were implemented to protect and maintain a healthy community.
- A registered nurse in New Zealand is responsible for improving the health outcomes for Māori, as well as being informed and responsive to all cultural and ethnic groups.

Self-test questions

1. You are asked the following question in a job interview or during your clinical placement: 'How will you implement the principles of the Treaty of Waitangi into your nursing practice?' How would you answer this?
2. Consider your own cultural background and practices. Would any of these need to be acknowledged and perhaps adapted in order to practise in a culturally safe manner in New Zealand?
3. When planning and implementing nursing care for your Māori client, what 'tapu' considerations first need to be identified in order not to offend?
4. When caring for a Māori client who has died, what key cultural safety practices do you need to be aware of? (You may need to refer to your local healthcare institution's policy and procedure guidelines to answer this question completely.)
5. Review the key terms and any other new vocabulary, terms and abbreviations from this chapter, and then update your 'Language list' (R2) on the CD Part 3—Reader resources.
6. Answer the 'Learning objectives' at the start of this chapter as if they were examination questions.

98

Chapter highlights at the end of each chapter provide a brief summary of the key points addressed in the chapter.

Self-test questions enable you to revise the topic. The questions with a number followed by 'a' (e.g. 3a) are for readers in Australia; the questions with a number followed by 'b' (e.g. 3b) are for readers in New Zealand; and those questions with plain numbers only (e.g. 7) are for all readers.

Sometimes, a question will require that you locate and read a journal article and complete an 'Article summary sheet'. The 'Article summary sheet' (R1) is located on the CD Part 3—Reader resources. This activity is to assist your ability to locate, understand and use current research in your studies and work. Nurses in Australia and New Zealand are expected to have up-to-date knowledge about nursing, and to regularly read professional journals.

There is one question in all chapters that requires you to review all new vocabulary, terms, expressions and abbreviations, and then to update your 'Language list'. The 'Language list' (R2) is located on the CD Part 3—Reader resources. This activity is to assist your language development.

There is one question in all chapters that requires you to review the 'Learning objectives' at the start of the chapter. This is a useful activity for checking that you understand the chapter content.

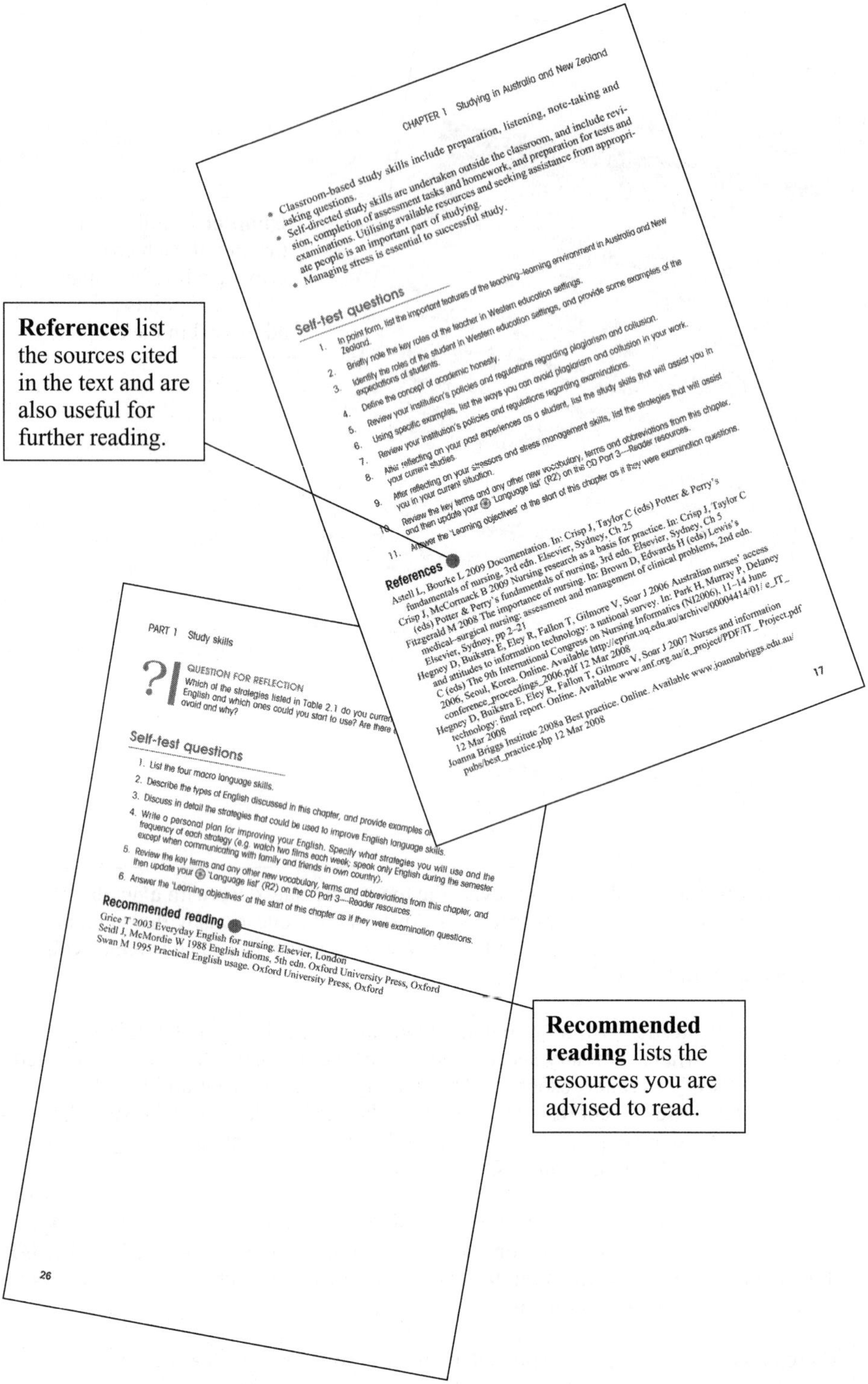
References list the sources cited in the text and are also useful for further reading.
Recommended reading lists the resources you are advised to read.

Acknowledgments

I would like to thank the following people whose contribution to this work is deeply appreciated:

- the team at Elsevier for their support, advice, professionalism, and for making this book a reality: Debra Gooley, Sabrina Chew, Helena Klijn, Eleanor Cant, Andreea Heriseanu, Ruth Matheson, Elinor Heard, Debbie Lee, who first invited me to write this text, and Sam McCulloch for her assistance at the start of this project
- Gill Srymgeour, for acting as the New Zealand content consultant and writing Chapter 6—her expert advice, support and wisdom have contributed significantly to this project
- Anna-Chur Hansen and Taryn Elliott for writing Chapter 8, and providing the content for the CD Part 1—Audio, 'Pronunciation of colloquialisms' (A1)—their generosity and willingness to share their earlier work is gratefully acknowledged
- The author gratefully acknowledges Austin Health, Heidelberg, Melbourne, Victoria, for permission to reproduce the hospital documents on the CD accompanying this book, and the assistance of Sue Thorpe in obtaining them
- Michelle Campbell for writing the foreword of this book
- Fabian Fitzgerald, Sound Engineer, Armstrong Studios
- Rob Fallon and John Hally for their participation in the recording of the CD
- my family, dearest friends and colleagues for their interest in and support of my work
- my parents, John and Aileen, whose love, support and practical assistance with child care is, as always, much appreciated, and
- Joe, my husband, and Xavier, our beautiful son, for their love, support, patience and encouragement throughout this process, and always.

Reviewers

I also gratefully acknowledge the following reviewers for their feedback and contribution to this work:

Cherry Campbell BSc DipN NZRN MHSc
Bachelor of Nursing Site Coordinator, Mokoia, School of Nursing and Health Studies—Te Puna Whai Ora, Waiariki Institute of Technology—Whare Takiura, Rotorua, New Zealand

Joo Lee RN BHSc (Nursing) PGDipAdvaN (Clinical Ed) MNS
Lecturer, School of Nursing, Faculty of Health and Behavioural Sciences, Deakin University, Victoria

Jennifer Hardy RN RM BSc MHP Ed PhD
Senior Lecturer, School of Nursing (NSW/ACT), Faculty of Health Sciences, Australian Catholic University

Patricia Josipovic RN DipAppSci (Nursing) EdBAppSc (Nursing) MEd (Research) RCNA
Head of School, School of Health, Faculty of Workforce Development, Victoria University

Ann Bride RN BSocSci, Masters (Nursing) Applied, Member of College of Nurses Aotearoa/New Zealand
Nurse Lecturer, Programme Coordinator—Bachelor of Nursing, Western Institute of Technology at Taranaki, New Zealand

About the author

Bernadette Hally RN DipAppSc (Nursing) BAppSc (Nursing) Dip Natural Therapy MEd MRCNA has worked as a clinician, clinical teacher, lecturer, nurse manager and consultant in a range of settings. Most recently, she has been a lecturer at the Australian Catholic University, St Patrick's Campus, Melbourne. She has been the Clinical Programs Co-ordinator (return to practice and graduate nurse programs) at a major metropolitan hospital in Melbourne, and a Manager/Nurse Consultant in International Education, researching overseas nurses' educational needs, and presenting to nurses in Malaysia and Singapore.

Her special interests are complementary therapies in nursing, international nursing, clinical education and competency development.

Bernadette has extensive experience working with international students in both tertiary and clinical settings, and is committed to assisting international nurses to meet nursing competency standards.

Contributors

Gill Scrymgeour RN BHSc (Nursing) (Auckland Institute of Technology) PGDipHSc (Advanced Nursing) MHSc (First Class Honours) University of Auckland (consultant for the New Zealand content and Chapter 6, 'Cultural safety in New Zealand nursing practice'): Gill Scrymgeour is the Programme Coordinator and senior lecturer of the Certificate in Contemporary New Zealand Nursing Practice (CCNZNP) at the Nursing School at the Eastern Institute of Technology, Hawke's Bay, New Zealand. The CCNZNP is a competency-based assessment program for international registered nurses seeking New Zealand registration and for New Zealand nurses returning to practice after a period of 5 years. Gill is also the Course Coordinator and Senior Lecturer of a Bachelor of Nursing paper ('Adolescent & Young Adult') and a postgraduate/Master of Nursing paper ('Advancing Specialty Practice'), and the Clinical Arts & Technology Centre Coordinator.

Dr Anna Chur-Hansen PhD (Chapter 8, 'Informal language in healthcare'; content for CD Part 1—Audio, 'Pronunciation of colloquialisms' (A1)): Associate Professor Anna Chur-Hansen is Deputy Head of the Discipline of Psychiatry at the University of Adelaide. She is a Registered Psychologist. Her primary role as an academic is to teach medical students, but she also teaches in nursing, health sciences and psychology. Her research focuses on health professional education. She is a Fellow of HERDSA (Higher Education Research and Development Society of Australasia), and a recipient of an inaugural Carrick Citation for her contributions to the health professional education literature.

Dr Taryn Elliott PhD (Chapter 8, 'Informal language in healthcare'; content for CD Part 1—Audio, 'Pronunciation of colloquialisms' (A1)): Dr Taryn Elliott graduated with a PhD in Psychology from the University of Adelaide in 2007 and has an interest in education research. Taryn has worked as an education researcher with the Adelaide to Outback GP Training Program (A2O) since 2004. During this time, she has overseen the growth of the International Medical Graduates (IMG) Fellowship Support Program, which assists doctors from overseas, who are recruited to rural areas of need to attain their GP Fellowship. Her other roles at A2O include Registrar-related project coordination, and educational research and evaluation. Part of this has seen her working on a project to assess and improve communication and language skills in GP Registrars and IMG doctors.

PART 1

Study skills

CHAPTER 1

Studying in Australia and New Zealand

'Studying here is very different from my country . . . here I must take responsibility for my learning, and also plagiarism is a big issue. In the past, I thought that if I used somebody's work, even if I did not use references, it was an honour to them!'

Jocelyn, India

CHAPTER OUTLINE

LEARNING OBJECTIVES

1. Briefly describe the nurse education environments relevant to students in Australia or New Zealand.
2. Discuss the roles of the teacher and the student in Australian or New Zealand nurse education settings.
3. Provide some examples of how students can maximise their learning opportunities (related to the roles of the teacher and student).

4. Discuss in detail the concepts of plagiarism and collusion.
5. Describe specific strategies a student could use to avoid plagiarism and collusion.
6. Describe in detail key strategies for maximising study skills.
7. Identify some stress management strategies for international students.

Key terms (are in bold in the text)

- academic honesty
- cheating
- clinical placement
- clinical practice guidelines
- clinical reasoning
- closed-book examination
- collusion
- computerised health records
- critical thinking
- electronic health records
- evidence-based nursing
- evidence-based practice (EBP)
- examination/test preparation
- information literacy
- information technology (IT)
- intellectual property
- Joanna Briggs Institute (JBI)
- lectures
- listening skills
- note-taking
- open-book examination
- personal digital assistants (PDAs)
- plagiarism
- practical classes
- preparation
- pre-reading
- principle-based learning
- principle-based teaching
- problem-based learning (PBL)
- reflection
- revision
- self-directed learning (SDL)
- self-directed study
- simulators
- study skills
- systematic review
- tutorials

To study in another country—particularly one where the language is different from your own—can be challenging. To succeed in your studies you will need a clear understanding of the teaching–learning environments and approaches in Australian and New Zealand nurse education. This includes the role expectations of teachers and students. One very important concept in Western education is academic honesty and students are required to abide by the relevant regulations at their teaching institutions. In addition, you will need to be motivated and conscientious in your study and have effective study skills, both in the classroom and at home.

Understanding the teaching–learning environment

It is important to understand the teaching–learning environment and some of the approaches to teaching–learning that will influence and impact on your experience of studying in Australia or New Zealand. It is particularly important to understand the roles of the teacher and the student within these contexts. One of the expectations of students is academic honesty. Ideas about academic honesty vary between cultures, particularly with respect to plagiarism and collusion. It is critical that you have a sound understanding of these concepts and how to avoid them in your studies.

Teaching–learning modes

While you might be enrolled in a program or some subjects that have been specifically tailored to meet your needs as an international student or an international nurse, it is important to remember that you will be expected to meet the same course requirements as local students—by successfully completing standard subjects and **clinical placement** requirements—and that you will need to meet the same requirements for registration as any other nurse.

Depending on your previous experiences as a student, you might find the classroom settings in Australia and New Zealand quite different. If you are studying at a university or polytechnic, you will find that **lectures** normally involve the lecturer addressing a large group, possibly up to a few hundred students. This may provide you with little opportunity for class participation. **Tutorials** are much smaller and students are expected to participate in class discussions and activities (which could include debates, role plays, small group work, case studies or presentations).

Nursing courses also include **practical classes** where students have the opportunity to learn and practise clinical nursing skills. In many places you will have the opportunity to use **simulators**, also sometimes called models, mannequins or 'dummies'. These are often used in practical classes for teaching and learning specific skills, such as basic life support.

In nursing subjects, the lectures, tutorials and practical classes often address the same topic in a different way. For example, following the lecture on the nursing care of patients with gastrointestinal disorders, the tutorial class might involve small groups of students working through a case study of a patient having gastric surgery and the practical class might be nasogastric tube insertion and management.

Teaching–learning methods and skills

Principle-based learning, problem-based learning (PBL), critical thinking, clinical reasoning and **evidence-based practice (EBP)** are very highly valued in Western nursing education, and students are expected to use them to assess clinical situations, identify the patient's problem and propose appropriate interventions (or care) to address the problems and to evaluate the interventions. (This is known as the nursing process and is addressed in Chs 11 and 13.) In addition, students are expected to be self-directed, able to reflect on their learning and have information literacy skills, in both the education and practice settings.

Problem-based learning (PBL)

Some approaches to teaching–learning, which might be new to you, include **problem-based learning (PBL)**. This involves students being given scenarios or case studies and requires the use of critical thinking and clinical reasoning skills to identify the problems and develop possible solutions. It requires students to identify and address their learning needs in the process (McLoughlin & Darvill 2007, Students On-line in Nursing and Integrated Curricula (SONIC) Project 2005).

Critical thinking

Critical thinking is a complex process involving a combination of high-level skills, including interpretation, analysis, evaluation, inference, explanation and reflection (Facione 1990 in Jones 2009 Ch 14). In nursing practice three levels of critical thinking have been identified: basic, complex and commitment (Kataoka-Yahiro & Saylor 1994). The use of language is considered to be an essential component of critical thinking, as the ability to use both is interrelated (Jones 2009 Ch 14). 'Critical thinking requires a framing of one's thoughts' (Jones 2009 Ch 14), and the nurse must also be able to use language to communicate clearly, and thus demonstrate critical thinking. English language development is therefore essential for international nurses and nursing students. (Chs 2, 10, 11 and 13 address aspects of communication and clinical practice in detail.)

Clinical reasoning

Clinical reasoning requires the application of specific clinical knowledge in problem solving and decision making, and is an example of the complex or commitment levels of critical thinking. Clinical reasoning also requires using nursing research as a basis for practice.

Evidence-based practice (EBP)

Evidence-based practice (EBP) is a process involving the synthesis of research about a topic (which when presented together is referred to as a **systematic review** of the research), the development of **clinical practice guidelines** (Joanna Briggs Institute 2008a), the implementation of the guidelines into practice and the evaluation of the outcomes (Crisp & McCormack 2009 Ch 5, Fitzgerald 2008 pp 12–13). When applied to nursing, EBP is referred to as **evidence-based nursing** and is 'the combination of individual clinical or professional expertise with the best available external evidence to produce practice that is most likely to lead to a positive outcome for a client or patient' (Joanna Briggs Institute 2008b).

EBP and evidence-based nursing are more than simply using research findings in practice, and you need to be able to access systematic reviews and clinical practice guidelines for your study. For Australian and New Zealand nurses and nursing students, the **Joanna Briggs Institute (JBI)** is an excellent resource, and it is recommended that you review its website, listed in the 'Recommended reading' at the end of the chapter (Joanna Briggs Institute 2008).

Principle-based teaching and principle-based learning

Principle-based teaching and **principle-based learning** are important in nursing, particularly as they relate to clinical skills. Clinical skills are usually taught according to principles, and this means that the student learns key principles associated with the skill, and then applies those principles to the actual performance of the skill. For example, to competently perform the clinical skills involved in wound management, the student would need to have learned the principles of asepsis and the principles of wound management. These principles would be specifically applied in assessing the wound, selecting the appropriate type of dressing material, planning the frequency of dressing changes and performing the dressing. This is quite a different approach from simply learning the sequence of steps involved in doing a wound dressing.

It is also important to note that just 'doing' a skill is not considered the same as being competent at a skill. Competence in clinical skills requires theoretical knowledge (related to the skill) and contextual knowledge (of the patient), as well as psychomotor skills to perform or 'do' the clinical skill. (See the discussion about competence in clinical skills in Chs 5, 12 and 13.)

Self-directed learning (SDL)

Self-directed learning is also a term with which you will become familiar as you study in Australia or New Zealand. Students are expected to take responsibility for their own learning and organise their own study. It is also expected that students will extend their learning beyond what is taught in the classroom. This can be achieved through completing set tasks, such as assignments, and by extensive reading (especially of texts and journals).

Reflection

Reflection is another aspect of self-directed learning that is used in nursing education, and is considered important in promoting professional development (Fitzgerald 2008 p 11, Jones 2009 Ch 14). It is possible that in your course you will be required to maintain a reflective journal—of your experiences, thoughts, feelings and actions. (Chs 12 and 13 address the concept of reflection as a nursing competency and reflection during clinical practice.)

Information literacy

Globally, **information technology (IT)** has had a significant impact on health, with health-related information readily accessible by most people (McMurray 2009 Ch 6). It is widely accepted that nurses require **information literacy** skills and that these skills are becoming increasingly important for all nurses.

Recent research has identified that nurses use information technology for a variety of purposes, including clinical practice, professional development activities, and management and administrative tasks (Hegney et al 2006, Hegney et al 2007). Clinical practice activities, such as documenting in **electronic health records**, which are also known as **computerised health records**, accessing results and patient records, and retrieving the information to support EBP all require IT skills. The use of **personal digital assistants (PDAs)** is also becoming more common in clinical nursing care.

Increasingly, professional development activities can be completed using electronic resources, and electronic records of professional development are required for nurses' portfolios (as discussed in Chs 5 and 14). Nurses working in management, administration and education are expected to be information literate. Important administrative and management tasks, such as rostering and staff allocation, also depend on IT (Astell & Bourke 2009 Ch 25, Fitzgerald 2008 p 14, Hegney et al 2006, Hegney et al 2007 pp 43–8). Similarly, students need to be information literate to research information, prepare and submit assignments, and participate in clinical experiences.

Role of the teacher

It is very important that you understand some beliefs about education from a Western cultural perspective. The word 'education' comes from the Latin words *educare* meaning to nourish or raise, and *ducere* meaning to lead. In this sense the teacher leads the student to new ideas, knowledge and ways of thinking, and does not simply tell the student information to be memorised. The teacher is responsible for ensuring that the course content is addressed, according to the accredited curriculum (as discussed in Ch 4), for directing students in their learning, and also for creating a positive learning environment where students are challenged, inspired and encouraged to share in the teaching and learning.

While it is reasonable to expect that your teachers are very knowledgeable about the subject area and competent in their teaching, they cannot know everything and will not be perfect. It is not considered impolite to ask your teacher questions or discuss the subject matter with your teacher (in fact this is actively encouraged). This is discussed later in this chapter.

Role of the student

As a student in Australia or New Zealand you will be expected to share the responsibility for your learning. This does not mean that your teachers will not assist you—rather that you are an important part of the process. Learning is an active process, and not a passive one. Even an excellent teacher cannot 'force' or make a student learn; the student needs to be motivated, conscientious and actively involved. The first step is to recognise that the responsibility for teaching–learning is shared by the teacher and the student.

You will be responsible for identifying your goals and learning needs, and for implementing strategies to assist you to meet your goals and needs, in consultation with your teachers where necessary. This is not as difficult as it sounds, but it might take you a little while to feel confident in doing so. Do not wait for your teacher to identify that you did not understand what was taught in class. If you do not seek assistance, as soon as possible, your difficulties might not be recognised until the topic is formally assessed (by assignment or examination) and then it could be too late to address your learning needs.

For example, if you experience difficulties understanding a topic, such as postoperative care or becoming competent in a skill, such as drug calculations, you will need to take action. You could do further reading using the resources you have been using in your course (e.g. the relevant sections on postoperative care in your medical–surgical nursing text) or complete further exercises (e.g. drug calculations). Ask your teacher questions in class or make an appointment to see your teacher. Specifically ask your teacher to recommend further work to help you. Do not be discouraged, even if you feel nervous doing this—it is all part of being an adult learner, and is actively encouraged in Western education.

In general, students are responsible for the grades they receive in their subjects. This does not mean that the teacher does not have a responsibility to assist the students, but the students' approach to study, along with their ability, have a significant influence on their subject results. This means that you can do many positive things to help you to achieve your study goals.

In classroom settings in Australia and New Zealand, students are encouraged to actively participate in many classes—and you will be expected to do so. This means that you will need to be prepared to answer questions, join discussions, work in small groups, participate in class presentations and ask questions. Make an effort to share your knowledge and experiences, particularly about nursing in your country. This way your teacher and other students also learn from you. This can be very difficult at first, but will become easier with practice. (The section on 'Study skills' in this chapter discusses in detail the strategies for maximising your learning opportunities.)

QUESTION FOR REFLECTION

How do teaching–learning, the role of the teacher and the role of the student in Australia and New Zealand compare to your previous experiences as a student in your country?

Academic honesty

Academic honesty refers to the integrity and truthfulness expected of students in relation to their studies. It is an expectation your teachers, teaching institutions and professional colleagues have of you, as a student. Your teaching institution will have policies and regulations about academic honesty in its handbook. All students are required to demonstrate academic honesty, and this expectation is no different for international students.

It is possible that some of the Western cultural understandings related to academic honesty will be quite new to you, or that the practices associated with ensuring academic honesty are different from those you have previously experienced as a student.

Essentially, the notion of academic honesty is based on the Western perspective of **intellectual property**. Intellectual property refers to someone's ideas and work (regardless of whether the work is published or not and whether or not it is copyright). For example, the lecture notes written by a nursing lecturer are the intellectual property of the lecturer. In Australia and New Zealand there are laws to protect intellectual property.

In Australian and New Zealand academic settings, any unauthorised use of other people's work—ideas, notes and publications—is considered to be stealing.

Plagiarism refers to the use of someone else's work without reference to that person. For example, if you copy a sentence from a text or journal and include it in your essay without quotation marks and referencing, you will have plagiarised. If you do not copy the sentence exactly, but include the ideas without referencing, you still will have plagiarised. In Australia and New Zealand using other people's work in this way is not considered to be a compliment or sign of respect to the original author, as it is in some countries. It is considered 'stealing' someone's intellectual property and is academically dishonest. The penalties for plagiarism depend on the institution, but range from failing the task or the subject, to being expelled from the institution.

Collusion refers to working with someone to complete an academic task (or having them do it for you) when you are required to submit your own work. For example, if you are required to write an essay and you ask a friend to do some of the work for you, you will have colluded with the other person. Collusion is a form of cheating and is deceptive, as the work submitted is assumed to be solely your own work and not (partially or fully) the work of another person. The penalties for collusion depend on the institution, but range from failing the task or the subject to being expelled from the institution.

Cheating is generally universally understood, but the degree to which it is practised and tolerated does vary. In Australia and New Zealand, the expectation of academic honesty does not make allowances for any student to cheat in any manner or under any circumstances or on any occasion. For example, taking notes into a **closed-book examination** (when this is not allowed) or taking additional materials into an **open-book examination** (apart from the notes, texts or other items allowed) is cheating and breaches the requirement for academic honesty. The presence of unauthorised material in an examination is considered a breach of academic honesty, even if you do not consult the material. The penalties for cheating depend on the institution, but range from failing the task or the subject to being expelled from the institution.

It is very important for you to understand that you will be expected to meet the requirements of academic honesty. You are responsible for being familiar with the policies or regulations about this concept at your teaching institution. Ignorance is not an acceptable excuse. You will also be expected to be able to reference correctly, using the style required at your institution. Remember to seek assistance from your teachers or other appropriate support staff if you are unsure about any matter related to academic honesty.

?

QUESTION FOR REFLECTION

How is the requirement for academic honesty in Australia and New Zealand different from the expectations of students in your country?

Study skills

In your nursing studies, you will experience a variety of learning opportunities—in the classroom and during clinical placements. It is very important that you maximise your opportunities to learn, both in the classroom and in your home-based study. (The learning skills you will need for clinical placement are discussed in detail in Chs 12 and 13.)

You will notice that the **study skills** strategies recommended in this chapter focus on developing key language skills—reading, writing, listening, comprehension and speaking. In addition, two skills required by all students are organisation and time management. You will find a 'Study skills checklist' (R3), a 'Sample subject organisation folder' (R4) and a 'Sample study planner' (R5) on the CD Part 3—Reader resources. Use these to help you develop your study skills.

In class

The learning strategies you use in class will help you to make the best use of your time at your teaching institution. Preparing for class, improving your listening skills in class, developing excellent note-taking skills—during class and when doing revision—and developing your confidence in asking questions in class will significantly assist you in your study.

Preparation

The first step in effective classroom-based learning is **preparation**. This means that you should attend the information or orientation sessions at your institution, and read the materials you receive prior to the commencement of your course. If you have specific subject information, also read this before the first class. Use your bilingual or medical–nursing dictionary to learn the definitions of words, terms or expressions that are new to you, and update your 'Language list' (R2) on the CD Part 3—Reader resources. After reading these materials, it is possible that you will feel overwhelmed. Remind yourself that this is quite normal. Write a list of questions to ask on your first day, so you can clarify your initial concerns.

After you have commenced your course, it is important to be prepared for every class. Make sure that you know the topics for the day's classes, do any **pre-reading** prescribed by your teacher or any preparation work you have been asked to do, and take all of the materials you need to class. If you have homework or assessment tasks due, they should be completed and submitted on time. When preparing for class, always write a list of questions to ask in class.

Listening

Listening in a second language requires enormous levels of concentration, and the subject matter might be new to you as well. Improving your English language skills (as discussed in Ch 2) will significantly improve your **listening skills**. During class, students can feel very overwhelmed. Keep reminding yourself that this happens to everyone, and with sound study skills you will develop confidence and soon feel much more comfortable in class. At first, you might find that you hear what is being said, but find it difficult to really listen (which means hearing and understanding). It is easier to listen if you have first read about the topic; therefore, it is very important to come to class well prepared, especially having read any relevant material. Ask your teacher if class notes are available prior to the class, and read them thoroughly and check the meaning of all new vocabulary before you attend the class. Write a list of questions to take to class.

In some cases, lectures are available for viewing or listening via the university website, after the class. It might be possible for you to tape-record lectures, but you need to check your institution's policy on tape-recording lectures and you *must* obtain permission from the lecturer on each occasion before doing so. It might be illegal to tape people without their knowledge.

Taking notes

Note-taking during class is an essential study skill. Taking notes in a second language is quite difficult, and improving your English language skills (as discussed in Ch 2) will significantly improve your note-taking skills. Always try to make a note of the key information, and do not attempt to write every word your teacher is saying. This is important because, firstly, it will be impossible for you to keep up and, secondly, your notes might not make much sense to you after class, unless you have understood the meaning of the topic.

Once again, being familiar with the topic before class, by preparing well, will help your understanding of the topic and, thus, your note-taking. If possible, add your own notes to printed class notes, and use point form where possible. These strategies will save you time and allow you more time to listen during the class.

During class—and also when revising your notes—use a highlighter pen or write a large question mark (or other symbol) to note any information that is confusing for you or about which you would like further information. You can then formulate questions to ask.

Asking questions

In Australia and New Zealand, teachers *expect* students to ask questions and raise discussion points about the topic. It is not considered impolite to ask questions. If you are concerned that you might sound too rude or challenging, you could preface your query with, 'Could I please ask you a question?' or 'Could you please explain . . .?' If you do not ask any questions, your teacher will assume that you understand the topic.

Often teachers will ask students if they have any questions at the end of class, or after explaining an idea or topic. Most teachers will strongly encourage you to raise your hand or simply speak up and ask questions during class. Make an effort to ask questions during class and do not save all of your questions to ask a teacher via email, telephone or during an appointment. Talking in class helps everyone to learn. Even though this might be unfamiliar to you and can be quite difficult at first, every teacher will tell you that students frequently have the same questions and teachers are often asked the same question by many students after class, when it could have been answered once in class . . . if someone had asked. Remember that the more often you speak in class and practise your English, the easier it will become.

It is recommended that you write a list of questions while you are preparing for class (when pre-reading notes and other information), while note-taking during class, and while revising notes after class. Take your lists of questions to your classes, but remember that you might need to ask your questions during a tutorial class if there is not an opportunity to do so during a lecture.

Self-directed study

Developing excellent study habits and **self-directed study** skills requires motivation and discipline. It is essential to study in your own time. If you check the hours allocated for most subjects each semester, you will note that the hours exceed the number of hours of classes. For example, if the hours for the subject are 120 and you have 30 hours of contact time (lectures, tutorials and practical classes), it is expected that you will complete 90 hours of self-study. This includes class preparation, revision, completing assessment tasks and homework, and studying for tests and examinations. It is important to plan your time so you can complete the study required for all of your subjects. Use the ◉ 'Sample study planner' (R5), on the CD Part 3—Reader resources, to help you.

Revision

Revision of class content needs to occur in your own time. Revision is much easier if you have collated the materials for each subject in an organised manner. Use the ◉ 'Sample subject organisation folder' (R4), on the CD Part 3—Reader resources, to assist you.

It is important to read over your class notes soon after the class. Add details to your notes, from texts or other sources, if you feel that further information is required. It is essential to clarify anything that is unclear to you at this stage. Often it is necessary to understand one topic before understanding the next topic. Do not wait until examinations are scheduled to do this. Write a list of questions for each subject using the list of questions section on the ◉ 'Sample subject organisation folder' (R4) on the CD Part 3—Reader resources.

When you have completed all the required reading, questions and self-test activities related to the topic, and feel confident that you have a sound understanding of the topic, make summary notes. You can use lists, charts, diagrams and colour coding to assist your memory. These should form the basis of your test or examination preparation, and can be completed well in advance.

Completing assessment tasks and homework

When you need to complete homework tasks or an assessment item (such as an essay, a class presentation or a poster), one of the most important things is to commence and complete the work on time. If you plan your time carefully, you will not need to rush the night before the task is due, or be late submitting the task. Both of these actions could affect your grade.

Start work on the task as soon as possible. Remember that because you are not working in your first language, it will probably take you longer to read, comprehend and understand the literature. Allow yourself 'spare' time.

Always ensure that you understand the task. Check the questions being asked, the type of assignment (such as case study, short answer, essay, report, survey) and any special requirements, including the word limit, format and due date. Carefully read all instructions about the task and ensure you clearly understand the marking guide. Use a highlighter pen or underline key words in the assignment question and make sure you are clear about the meaning of directives such as 'list', 'identify', 'describe', 'explain', 'discuss', 'compare', 'contrast', 'critically analyse' and 'provide rationales'. Always complete the task exactly as required.

It is essential that you reference correctly, using the style required by your institution. If you experience difficulties with referencing, speak to your teacher or the relevant support person at the institution, well before the task is due. See the 'Completing assessment tasks and homework' section of the 'Study skills checklist' (R3) on the CD Part 3—Reader resources.

Plan to complete the task well before it is due for submission. This will allow you time to check your work carefully, and amend it where necessary. Remember that poor organisation and time management are *not* reasons to justify asking for an extension of the due date.

It is recommended that you retain a hard copy or photocopy of your completed assessment task, even if submitted electronically. It is not sufficient to have only electronic copies of your work. In some places, you are required to do this, and you must be able to produce a hard copy for marking, in the event that the institution loses the work. Sometimes a receipt is given to students as verification of task submission, and students must be able to produce this on request. In many places, students must submit a declaration of honesty with their completed assessment tasks, stating that they have not plagiarised, colluded or cheated.

Examination/test preparation

Good **examination/test preparation** reduces stress. Ideally, preparation for examinations and tests should start when you revise the topics studied, clarify any questions and make your summary notes (see the information above about revision).

Ask your teacher for further clarification of anything that you do not understand. Try to do this as soon as possible in your examination preparation.

Many teachers provide examination preparation information about the subject. Listen and take notes at these sessions. It is essential to know the content being examined. If you are unsure, clarify the scope of the examination—that is, which topics are being tested (often it is the entire subject content). Check the format (multiple-choice questions, short-answer questions, essays, case studies, listening comprehension), duration and special conditions of the examination (such as open book, closed book and whether the use of bilingual dictionaries is permitted).

It is often very beneficial to study with a partner or in a small group, but make sure that this is helpful for you and is not distracting you or preventing you from progressing in your studies. It is useful for group members to 'test' each other, by preparing sample questions or using questions from lecture objectives, texts or past examination papers.

If you have access to previous examination papers, practise doing these papers under examination conditions. Ensure that you practise good time management. Remember to take note of the marks allocated for each section or question and allocate appropriate time for each question.

If there is reading time in the examination, use it to read the paper carefully (you will not be allowed to write *at all* during this time). During the examination, take note of the marks allocated for each section or question and allocate appropriate time for each question. When you are permitted to commence writing, use a highlighter pen or underline key words in the questions and ensure that you understand the directives often used in test and examination questions, such as 'list', 'identify', 'describe', 'explain', 'discuss', 'compare', 'contrast', 'critically analyse' and 'provide rationales'.

It is your responsibility to comply with the examination regulations and the academic honesty policies and regulations at your institution. Read these policies and regulations, and check with your teachers if you are uncertain about any requirements. You should expect to provide your student identification card, pens and other equipment, such as a calculator (if allowed), for every examination. Do not take any unauthorised material into the examination room, such as books, notes or mobile telephones. If you are allowed to take bags and mobile telephones into the examination room, remember to turn off your mobile telephone, and if possible remove the SIM card before entering the examination room. Always check your institution's policy about bilingual dictionaries. You might need to have special permission to use a dictionary, and this should be arranged before the examination. See the 'Examination/test preparation' section of the 'Study skills checklist' (R3) on the CD Part 3—Reader resources.

Table 1.1 outlines the specific strategies for developing your study skills. Use these strategies and the 'Study skills checklist' (R3), the 'Sample subject organisation folder' (R4) and the 'Sample study planner' (R5), on the CD Part 3—Reader resources, to assist you.

TABLE 1.1 Strategies for developing your study skills

Organisation and time management	
Organise all subjects (see the 'Sample subject organisation folder' (R4) on the CD Part 3—Reader resources)	
Complete the study planner (see the 'Sample study planner' (R5) on the CD Part 3—Reader resources)	
In class	
Preparation	Pre-reading (prescribed material) Pre-reading (class notes) Update the 'Language list' (R2) on the CD Part 3—Reader resources List questions Other homework
Listening	Get permission for taping Practise listening (not just hearing)
Note-taking	Use point form Note main ideas List questions
Asking questions	Ask questions in class

TABLE 1.1 Strategies for developing your study skills—*cont'd*

Organisation and time management	
Self-directed study	

Revision	Read your notes
	List questions
	  Clarify all queries (extra reading, ask teacher)
	  Add details to notes
	  Summarise topic notes
	  Test yourself
	Completing assessment tasks and homework
	  Note due date
	  Check understanding of the task
	  Complete task
	    Reference correctly
	    Review work
	    Photocopy work
	Submit correctly

Examination/test preparation	Read examination/test policies and regulations
	Locate the examination timetable
	Clarify the examination/test details
	  Scope
	  Format
	  Duration
	  Special conditions
	  Date/time/location
	Clarify any queries about subject content
	Review own topic summary notes
	Complete past exams
	Study in a group

Seeking help	
The following people can help you with study skills:	Teachers Study skills advisors Tutors Other professionals (depending on issues—for example, speech pathologist, counsellor)

?

QUESTION FOR REFLECTION

In your previous experience as a student, how have you managed your studies and how could these skills assist you now?

Stress management

It is important for everyone to manage stress. All students can find studying very stressful at times, and for international students this can be compounded by homesickness, adjusting to a new culture, financial concerns and difficulties with language.

Good organisation and time management skills can assist students to manage their studies. In addition to healthy eating habits, including regular exercise, leisure and recreation time into your routine are essential for good health and stress management.

Having support from friends is particularly important if you are living away from your family. If you find living alone difficult, consider options such as sharing a house or living with a homestay family (the latter will also assist your language development if the family speaks English).

If you feel that you need assistance to manage stress, see the relevant person at your institution. Depending on your situation, it might be useful to talk with a counsellor, study skills advisor or one of your teachers.

QUESTION FOR REFLECTION

Reflect on the major stressors in your life, the strategies you currently use to manage stress and those you could adopt.

CHAPTER HIGHLIGHTS

- In the teaching–learning environment in Australia and New Zealand, nursing students will experience a variety of approaches, including principle-based teaching, problem-based learning and self-directed learning.
- The development of critical thinking and clinical reasoning skills is considered very important for nursing students.
- Critical thinking and clinical reasoning are applied to problem-based learning and evidence-based practice.
- Students are expected to reflect on their classroom and clinical learning experiences.
- Students and nurses are expected to develop skills in information literacy to support their study and practice.
- Teachers are expected to 'lead' the students, but are not solely responsible for the students' results.
- Students are expected to assume responsibility for their own learning, to be active participants in the teaching–learning process, to set and meet learning goals and to be self-directed in their approach to study.
- The concept of academic honesty is based on Western cultural understandings of intellectual property, and is expected of all students.
- In Australian and New Zealand academic settings, any unauthorised use of other people's work—ideas, notes and publications—is considered to be stealing.
- Plagiarism, collusion and cheating are considered serious offences within academic settings.
- Study skills are essential for academic success and focus on key language skills—reading, writing, listening, comprehension and speaking.

- Classroom-based study skills include preparation, listening, note-taking and asking questions.
- Self-directed study skills are undertaken outside the classroom, and include revision, completion of assessment tasks and homework, and preparation for tests and examinations. Utilising available resources and seeking assistance from appropriate people is an important part of studying.
- Managing stress is essential to successful study.

Self-test questions

1. In point form, list the important features of the teaching–learning environment in Australia and New Zealand.
2. Briefly note the key roles of the teacher in Western education settings.
3. Identify the roles of the student in Western education settings, and provide some examples of the expectations of students.
4. Define the concept of academic honesty.
5. Review your institution's policies and regulations regarding plagiarism and collusion.
6. Using specific examples, list the ways you can avoid plagiarism and collusion in your work.
7. Review your institution's policies and regulations regarding examinations.
8. After reflecting on your past experiences as a student, list the study skills that will assist you in your current studies.
9. After reflecting on your stressors and stress management skills, list the strategies that will assist you in your current situation.
10. Review the key terms and any other new vocabulary, terms and abbreviations from this chapter, and then update your 'Language list' (R2) on the CD Part 3—Reader resources.
11. Answer the 'Learning objectives' at the start of this chapter as if they were examination questions.

References

Astell L, Bourke L 2009 Documentation. In: Crisp J, Taylor C (eds) Potter & Perry's fundamentals of nursing, 3rd edn. Elsevier, Sydney, Ch 25

Crisp J, McCormack B 2009 Nursing research as a basis for practice. In: Crisp J, Taylor C (eds) Potter & Perry's fundamentals of nursing, 3rd edn. Elsevier, Sydney, Ch 5

Fitzgerald M 2008 The importance of nursing. In: Brown D, Edwards H (eds) Lewis's medical–surgical nursing: assessment and management of clinical problems, 2nd edn. Elsevier, Sydney, pp 2–21

Hegney D, Buikstra E, Eley R, Fallon T, Gilmore V, Soar J 2006 Australian nurses' access and attitudes to information technology: a national survey. In: Park H, Murray P, Delaney C (eds) The 9th International Congress on Nursing Informatics (NI2006), 11–14 June 2006, Seoul, Korea. Online. Available http://eprint.uq.edu.au/archive/00004414/01/ e_IT_conference_proceedings_2006.pdf 12 Mar 2008

Hegney D, Buikstra E, Eley R, Fallon T, Gilmore V, Soar J 2007 Nurses and information technology: final report. Online. Available www.anf.org.au/it_project/PDF/IT_ Project.pdf 12 Mar 2008

Joanna Briggs Institute 2008a Best practice. Online. Available www.joannabriggs.edu.au/pubs/best_practice.php 12 Mar 2008

Joanna Briggs Institute 2008b Evidence based nursing. Online. Available www.joannabriggs.edu.au/about/eb_nursing.php 12 Mar 2008
Jones B 2009 Critical thinking and nursing judgment. In: Crisp J, Taylor C (eds) Potter & Perry's fundamentals of nursing, 3rd edn. Elsevier, Sydney, Ch 14
Kataoka-Yahiro M, Saylor C 1994 A critical thinking model for nursing judgement. Journal of Nursing Education 33(8):351
McLoughlin M, Darvill A 2007 Peeling back the layers of learning: a classroom model for problem-based learning. Nurse Education Today 27(4):271–277
McMurray A 2009 Health and wellness. In: Crisp J, Taylor C (eds) Potter & Perry's fundamentals of nursing, 3rd edn. Elsevier, Sydney, Ch 6
Students On-line in Nursing and Integrated Curricula (SONIC) Project 2005 Problem based learning. Online. Available www.uclan.ac.uk/facs/health/nursing/sonic/PBL.htm 12 Mar 2008

Recommended reading

Joanna Briggs Institute 2008 Joanna Briggs Institute. Online. Available www.joannabriggs.edu.au 12 Mar 2008

CHAPTER 2

Improving your English

'English is one of the hardest things about studying here and I am worried about if my patients and colleagues will understand me, and if I can understand them. I always try to talk in English—even at home with my housemates. I must also try to do it when I am nervous—for example, answering the telephone using English.'

Miwa, Japan

CHAPTER OUTLINE

LEARNING OBJECTIVES

1. Briefly describe the English requirements for studying in Australia or New Zealand.
2. Describe the types of English used when living, studying and working in Australia or New Zealand.
3. Describe strategies to improve English language skills.
4. Develop a personal plan for developing English language skills.

Key terms (are in bold in the text)

academic English
general English
macro language skills
'nursing' English
professional English

As you will be aware, it can be very difficult to study in another country, particularly one where the language is different from your own. To succeed in your studies and work in Australia or New Zealand, you will need to be confident and competent in communicating in English.

English language proficiency testing

All international students and overseas trained nurses and midwives must meet minimum language requirements before being able to study or work in Australia or New Zealand. English proficiency testing addresses the four **macro language skills**. These skills are reading, writing, listening and speaking. Some tests focus on general language and do not specifically test that a person is prepared for academic study or professional work, while others are occupation specific. Certainly, the more proficient you are in **general English**, the easier it will be to develop **academic English** and **professional English** skills.

Although you will have already met the minimum language criterion for studying or working in Australia or New Zealand, most international students and nurses discover that considerably more work is needed for them to feel confident and competent in their general, academic and professional **'nursing' English** language skills. While this can seem overwhelming at first, it is important to remember that language skills can be developed, and there are many opportunities for doing so.

?

QUESTION FOR REFLECTION

How confident do you feel reading, writing, listening and speaking in English?

Types of English

In order to develop your English language skills, it is useful to consider the types of English you will need while living, studying and working in Australia or New Zealand. Apart from general formal and informal English language skills, you will also need to have excellent academic and formal and informal professional 'nursing' English language skills. Figure 2.1 outlines the types of English and some examples of each.

?

QUESTION FOR REFLECTION

Reflect on your ability to communicate using all of the types of English identified in Figure 2.1.

Improving your English

No matter how concerned you feel about your language proficiency, always remember that there are many things you can do to improve your English. Often students and international nurses forget that language development is effectively another subject to study, and requires time, practice and being actively engaged in the community. Living, studying and working in native English-speaking countries is the perfect opportunity to immerse yourself in English.

FIGURE 2.1 Types of English

Professional 'nursing' English—informal
Used for: communicating in all professional nursing settings.
Prerequisites: general (formal and informal), academic and professional 'nursing' English.
Examples: Patient uses health-related idioms and colloquialisms during admission interview.
Nurse uses health-related idioms and colloquialisms during verbal handover.

Professional 'nursing' English—formal
Used for: communicating in all professional nursing settings.
Prerequisite: general (formal and informal) and academic English.
Examples: Nurse uses 'nursing' English during verbal handover.
Nurse uses 'nursing' English when documenting in the nursing progress notes.

Academic English
Used for: communicating in academic settings and professional publications.
Prerequisite: general English.
Examples: The nursing assignment must be written using academic English.
A nursing journal article uses academic English.

General English—informal
Used for: communicating in everyday life.
Prerequisite: general English.
Examples: A local student is telling you about his weekend activities, and uses idioms and colloquialisms in the conversation.
You are reading a novel in which informal language is used.

General English
Used for: communicating in everyday life.
Prerequisite: basic English language skills.
Examples: A ticket inspector on the train asks to check your ticket.
You order a meal at a restaurant.

Use all of the available opportunities to develop your English language skills and do not avoid reading, writing, listening and speaking in English. This is very important, particularly if you always use your own language when at home. While it is natural to speak your first language with other students from your country, make it a habit to speak English as much as possible, and certainly whenever you are at university or work. This will help you—and your fellow students—improve your English.

As part of your normal daily activities, make an effort to speak with native English speakers (talk with shop assistants, your neighbours, other students or colleagues), listen to the radio and watch television programs and films (select the English soundtrack and use English subtitles as well, until you feel confident in your listening comprehension), read everything you see (newspapers, advertising material, signs, maps, posters), and write (emails, notes, letters) in English as much as possible.

If you can live with a local family under a homestay arrangement, this will help your English language development considerably. You will be readily engaged in normal English conversation on a daily basis and have access to English reading materials and other media. Ideally, living in a family could also be a form of support for you. If you do not live with local people or native speakers, ensure that you participate in the community—through a club, group or church.

Maintain a 'Language list' (R2) (on the CD Part 3—Reader resources) for all new vocabulary, expressions, medical and nursing terminology, jargon and abbreviations. Keep this document with you at all times and aim to learn at least one new word, term or expression every day.

For study and work, you need to be confident and competent in the English required. Attend any sessions at your teaching institution, workplace or in the community that are designed to assist your academic or professional English language skills. Ensure that you are well prepared for classes (do all pre-reading), and practise asking questions and participating in class discussions. Read extensively. This will also assist your writing skills and help your oral communication. Use the feedback you receive about your written work and improve your writing with each new task. Rehearse oral presentations and handovers to ensure you can be clearly understood by the audience. Seek assistance from a teacher, study skills advisor, English as a second language (ESL) tutor or other professional (such as a speech pathologist for pronunciation) to assist you to improve your English.

Expect to make mistakes. This is normal and is an important part of learning another language. Ask native speakers to help you to correct your mistakes. Specifically, ask them to correct your grammar, expressions and pronunciation during conversation.

It is a nursing competency requirement that you can communicate effectively in English. To be a safe and competent nurse and nursing student you *must* be able to communicate 'like a native English-speaking nurse'. (See Ch 5 for a detailed discussion of nursing competency standards and Ch 13 for information about the assessment of competency standards during clinical placements.) Your patients' safety depends on your ability to communicate well in English. Sometimes, students believe that activities such as reading newspapers, listening to the radio and watching television are too difficult or boring. Remember that local students and nurses—and your patients—can understand complex newspaper articles, radio broadcasts and the television news, so you need to be able to do so too.

Table 2.1 outlines some specific strategies for developing your English. Commit to using these ideas, and the strategies suggested for developing your verbal communication and documentation skills (in Chs 10 and 11), on a regular basis. Many can be included in your normal daily activities.

CHAPTER HIGHLIGHTS

- You will need to improve your English language skills beyond the minimum requirements for studying or working in Australia or New Zealand.
- You will need excellent (formal and informal) general, academic and (formal and informal) professional 'nursing' English language skills.
- Use every opportunity to improve your English language skills and do not avoid using English.
- Effective communication in English is a nursing competency requirement.
- Language skills—reading, writing, listening and speaking—can be improved using specific strategies.

TABLE 2.1 Strategies for improving your English

Types of English	Reading	Writing	Listening	Speaking
General English	Living, studying and working (even part-time) in an English-speaking country will help your language skills if you *actively* engage in the community. Consider joining a group or club, attending a church or doing volunteer or paid work.			
	Add all new vocabulary to your 'Language list' (R2) on the CD Part 3—Reader resources. Update the list daily.	Always check your grammar and spelling, and ask for feedback.	Listen . . . and understand. Check your understanding by discussing what you have heard.	Speak as much as possible, and ask people to correct your pronunciation. Speak slowly and clearly. See a speech pathologist or an ESL tutor for help with pronunciation if necessary.
Formal	Read the main newspapers or articles from the newspaper every day. Read your local community newspaper every week. Read novels. Read magazines.	Write letters, notes and email messages.	Have many conversations in English. Listen to local radio and watch films and television programs. Watch the news on television 5–7 nights per week. Watch current affairs programs on television. Watch films in English and use English subtitles as well. Live with a local homestay family.	Talk in English as often as possible with as many people as possible. Speak to your neighbours, local students or colleagues, and salespeople. Live with a local homestay family.
Informal	Read novels (by local authors).	Send text (SMS) messages via mobile telephones.	As above—where informal language is used	As above—where informal language is used
Academic English	*In addition* to the strategies for improving your general English:			
	Read journals. Read texts.	Attend all relevant academic skills sessions at your institution.	Tape lectures if permitted (or view/listen a second time if they are available online).	Record yourself speaking. Check your: • volume

(Continued)

TABLE 2.1 Strategies for improving your English—*cont'd*

Types of English	Reading	Writing	Listening	Speaking
Academic English—cont'd	Reading will improve your writing skills and your referencing.	Use point form for note-taking. Use spelling and grammar checks on your computer. See a teacher or a study skills advisor if you are having difficulties. Use dictionaries.	Use point form and note the main ideas (so you have more time to listen in class). Do pre-reading before class (so you have some idea of what to expect when listening).	• pace • pronunciation • clarity (of words and expressions), and • eye contact. For class presentations also: • have notes for reference (but *do not* read them) • practise your speech, using a mirror, and • practise with a friend or colleague.
Professional 'nursing' English	*In addition* to the strategies for improving your general English and academic English: Consider doing volunteer or paid work in the health or aged care sector. If you are an overseas registered nurse, you might be able to work as an unregistered personal carer before completing your studies.			
Formal	Read the documentation found in clinical settings. Update your 'Language list' (R2), on the CD Part 3—Reader resources, with medical and nursing jargon (see Ch 9).	Practise 'nursing writing' (see Ch 11). Ask a teacher or colleague to review a draft of your progress notes and other documentation.	Ask for information to be repeated if necessary. Restate key information you have heard (to ensure you have understood). Clarify all queries. Watch local television programs and listen to local radio programs with medical, nursing or health content (dramas, soap operas, documentaries, current affairs). Complete Part 7, 'Learning activities for use with CD'.	For handovers: • have notes for reference • use jargon appropriately, and • practise with a colleague or clinical teacher. For communicating in clinical settings: • use jargon appropriately, and • check that the person listening has understood you. Complete Part 7, 'Learning activities for use with CD'.

TABLE 2.1 Strategies for improving your English—*cont'd*

Types of English	Reading	Writing	Listening	Speaking
Informal	Review the list of expressions in Chapter 8.	Use abbreviations for your nursing handover notes.	Ask for an explanation of any expression you do not understand. Listen to the CD Part 1—Audio, 'Pronunciation of colloquialisms' (A1) and 'Pronunciation of phrasal verbs' (A2).	Have general conversations with nurses.

?

QUESTION FOR REFLECTION

Which of the strategies listed in Table 2.1 do you currently use regularly to improve your English and which ones could you start to use? Are there any strategies that you currently avoid and why?

Self-test questions

1. List the four macro language skills.
2. Describe the types of English discussed in this chapter, and provide examples of each.
3. Discuss in detail the strategies that could be used to improve English language skills.
4. Write a personal plan for improving your English. Specify what strategies you will use and the frequency of each strategy (e.g. watch two films each week; speak only English during the semester except when communicating with family and friends in own country).
5. Review the key terms and any other new vocabulary, terms and abbreviations from this chapter, and then update your 'Language list' (R2) on the CD Part 3—Reader resources.
6. Answer the 'Learning objectives' at the start of this chapter as if they were examination questions.

Recommended reading

Grice T 2003 Everyday English for nursing. Elsevier, London
Seidl J, McMordie W 1988 English idioms, 5th edn. Oxford University Press, Oxford
Swan M 1995 Practical English usage. Oxford University Press, Oxford

PART 2

Nursing in Australia and New Zealand

CHAPTER 3

Healthcare systems

'I can understand that I must know about Indigenous people. It is a big problem about their health—even in this country, which has so many good health services.'

Tam, Hong Kong

CHAPTER OUTLINE

LEARNING OBJECTIVES

1. Briefly describe the Australian or New Zealand population and demographics.
2. Discuss the Australian healthcare system or New Zealand health and disability system.
3. Describe the types of healthcare services in Australia or New Zealand.
4. Briefly compare the Western biomedical model of health with complementary or alternative therapies.
5. Describe the concerns associated with the health of Indigenous people in Australia or New Zealand.
6. Discuss the concept of registration for health professionals.
7. Define the types of health professionals in Australia and New Zealand.

Key terms (are in bold in the text)

Aboriginal
Accident Compensation Corporation (ACC) (NZ)
accident compensation scheme
acute care
alternative medicine/therapies
biomedical model
'bulk bill'
Charter of Patients Rights and Responsibilities (Aus)
Code of Health and Disability Services Consumers' Rights (NZ)
Commonwealth (Aus)
community care
complementary and alternative medicine (CAM)
complementary medicine/therapies
'cover'
District Health Boards (DHBs) (NZ)
federal
'gap'
Health and Disability Commission (HDC) (NZ)
Health and Disability Commissioner Act (NZ)
health cover
Health Practitioners Competence Assurance Act (HPCAA) (NZ)
holistic medicine/therapies
Indigenous
Māori
Medicare (Aus)
natural medicine/therapies
not-for-profit
'out-of-pocket' expense
premium
primary care
primary healthcare
Primary Health Organisations (PHOs) (NZ)
private health fund
professional board
rebate
registered
residential care
scheduled fee
secondary care
subacute care
tertiary care
the Crown (NZ)
the Special High Cost Treatment Pool (NZ)
Torres Strait Islanders (TSIs)
traditional medicine/therapies
Western medicine
(See also the list of health professionals in this chapter.)

To understand the healthcare systems in Australia and New Zealand, it is important to have a basic understanding of the populations, types of government, funding of healthcare, the main models of healthcare, healthcare services and the types of healthcare professionals in each country. It is also important to be aware of key issues in healthcare, particularly Indigenous health in both Australia and New Zealand.

Healthcare systems

The healthcare systems in Australia and New Zealand are generally considered to be of a very high standard. The governments in both countries are democratically elected, and healthcare is seen as very important by the citizens of Australia and New Zealand, and is a matter that is considered seriously when electing governments.

The Australian population and demographics

The Australian population is approximately 21.2 million (Australian Bureau of Statistics 2008), with approximately 61% of people living in large cities (Sydney, Melbourne, Brisbane, Perth and Adelaide) and almost 14% living in 13 smaller cities. Approximately 24% of the population lives in rural areas (with almost 60% of these people living in regional cities and towns). Less than 3% of the population lives in remote areas (Newton 2001).

The **Indigenous** population accounts for approximately 2.4% of the total population. Of these people, 90% are Aboriginal, 6% are Torres Strait Islanders and 4% are both. Approximately 50% of Indigenous people live in urban areas of New South Wales and Queensland, and 25% live in remote or very remote areas of Australia. In the Northern Territory, 29% of the population is Indigenous.

Approximately 24% of the Australian population was born overseas. People living in Australia come from over 200 countries. Approximately 53% of people born overseas are from Europe or the former USSR, approximately 24% are from Asian regions, and smaller proportions were born in Oceania and Antarctica (mainly from New Zealand), Africa and the Middle East, and the Americas (Australian Bureau of Statistics 2001).

The Australian healthcare system

The **Commonwealth** Department of Health and Aged Care is the Australian **federal** (which means national) government department responsible for healthcare in Australia. It has a 'leadership role in policy making and . . . national issues like public health, research and national information management' (Commonwealth Department of Health and Aged Care 2000 p 1).

Each state and territory also has its own health department that is 'primarily responsible for the delivery and management of public health services and for maintaining direct relationships with most healthcare providers, including the regulation of health professionals' (Commonwealth Department of Health and Aged Care 2000 p 1).

In addition, local governments in the states and territories provide some healthcare services to communities. Local governments are sometimes referred to as 'councils' or 'shires'.

The Commonwealth and state/territory governments share the funding for many healthcare services in Australia (see Fig 3.1).

Primary care, which is healthcare received in the community, not in hospitals, is provided by a range of health professionals, including doctors, nurses, allied health professionals, chiropractors, osteopaths, pharmacists and Chinese medicine practitioners.

The Australian healthcare system has public and private sectors offering a broad range of practitioners and services. In Australia, private and public health insurance coexist.

FIGURE 3.1 Overview of the Australian healthcare system and services

Level of government — **Government bodies and responsibilities**

Federal

Commonwealth Department of Health and Aged Care

Leadership:
Policy
Public health
Research
Information
Funding

Various sectors and portfolios, including the Office for Aboriginal and Torres Strait Islander Health (OATSIH)

State/territory

Health departments (variously named)

Management of public health services
Relationships with health professions
Regulation of health professions
Funding

Local

Councils/shires

Delivery of healthcare services in local area

Health services

Public
(Medicare)

Levels/degrees
Primary care—community
Secondary care—hospitals
Tertiary care—specialised doctors

Needs-based
Acute (e.g. medical-surgical, specialised)
Subacute (e.g. rehabilitation, palliative, interim)
Residential (e.g. aged, disability)
Community (e.g. aged care in home)

Health focus
Maternity
Mental health
Disability
Aged
Palliative
Indigenous
Chronic health condition (e.g. diabetes)
And others

Private
Natural therapies (some private health insurance companies provide refunds)

The public health insurance scheme is called **Medicare** (and is funded in part by the Australian taxation system). All eligible Australians can receive free healthcare in the public health system, including free medicines while in hospital. Patients using public hospitals cannot choose the doctor who will care for them; they will usually be cared for by a doctor who is employed by the hospital. People with Medicare entitlements can also receive reduced-cost medicines (which are purchased at pharmacies or chemist shops) through the Pharmaceutical Benefits Scheme (PBS) (Commonwealth Department of Health and Aged Care 2000).

After consulting a general practitioner (GP) or optometrist, people with Medicare entitlements also receive a refund (or **rebate**) after paying the bill for these services. If the bill is for the **scheduled fee** (which is like a recommended price), the patient will not be 'out of pocket', meaning the patient receives a full refund of the amount paid. Some doctors charge more than the scheduled fee, so the Medicare refund will only be for the scheduled fee. The patient's **'out-of-pocket' expense** is also referred to as the **'gap'**, meaning the difference between the scheduled fee and the fee actually charged.

In some cases, the practitioner does not bill the patient at all, but will **'bulk bill'** the government. This means that the practitioner sends the bills for many patients to the government, and the Medicare payment is paid directly to the practitioner. These practitioners charge only the scheduled fee.

Australians can choose to purchase private health insurance for a fee or **'premium'** directly from a private health insurance company, also known as a **private health fund**. Individuals or families can have private health insurance policies. This means that they can use private health services, and can avoid public hospital waiting lists for elective surgery by going to a private hospital, and have a choice of which doctors to engage in private hospitals. The patient then receives a refund for hospital or other non-hospital health services, including consultations and treatments by community-based natural therapists (such as chiropractors). Depending on the level of insurance, also called **'health cover'**, there may be 'out-of-pocket' expenses or 'gaps' if the practitioner or service charges the patient more than the insurance company will refund (i.e. more than the scheduled fee).

Rights and responsibilities for Australian healthcare consumers

While the Australian Commission on Safety and Quality in Health Care has recommended that Australia develops a national **Charter of Patients' Rights and Responsibilities** within the public health system, currently each state and territory in Australia has a separate charter. While there are some differences, they address the rights outlined in Table 3.1.

Australia has also developed a Private Patients' Hospital Charter that outlines what private patients can expect from doctors, hospitals and health insurance funds (Australian Government Department of Health and Ageing 2007). As far as patient rights regarding patient care, there are strong similarities to the rights contained in the charters developed for the public system.

The New Zealand population and demographics

There are approximately 4.26 million people in New Zealand (Statistics New Zealand 2008), with 75% of people living in the North Island. Approximately 71% of people live in major urban areas, 6.3% live in secondary urban areas, 8.45% live in minor urban areas and 14.3% live in rural centres and areas (Statistics New Zealand 2006a).

TABLE 3.1 Overview of the charters of patients' rights and responsibilities in Australia

Patients within the public health system have the right to: • access the public health system • free treatment and care within the public health system • quality care • be treated with respect • access personal medical records • healthcare information • participate in decision making, and to provide informed consent for treatment and procedures • participate in undergraduate education and research • confidentiality and privacy of medical and personal information • an interpreter if required, and • complain about healthcare.
Patients within the public health system have the responsibility to: • recognise the priorities and limitations of healthcare staff • communicate all relevant information • seek clarification if unsure of any matter related to their healthcare, and • respect staff, visitors and other patients.

Source: ACT Health 2007, Department of Health and Human Services Tasmania 2005, Department of Health South Australia 2005, Department of Health Western Australia 2004, Department of Human Services Victoria 2007, Health and Community Services Complaints Commission Northern Territory undated, New South Wales Health 2005, Queensland Health 2007.

The Māori population accounts for approximately 17.7% of the total population. Approximately 87% of Māori live in the North Island and approximately 24% of Māori live in Auckland (Statistics New Zealand 2006d).

Approximately 23% of the New Zealand population was born overseas. Of these, 28.6% were born in the United Kingdom and Ireland, and 28.6% were born in Asia (predominantly China) (Statistics New Zealand 2006e).

The New Zealand health and disability system

The national government in New Zealand is referred to as **the Crown**. Its Ministry of Health is the government department responsible for New Zealand's health and disability system. It provides 'national policy advice, regulation, funding, and monitoring the performance of agency' (New Zealand Ministry of Health 2003). There are 21 **District Health Boards (DHBs)**, which are responsible for 'providing, or funding the provision of health and disability services in their district' (New Zealand Ministry of Health 2003), as part of the implementation of the New Zealand Health Strategy and the New Zealand Disability Strategy.

In New Zealand, primary care is provided to members of the community by various healthcare professionals, and includes:

> . . . first level services such as general practice services [medical care provided by general practitioners], mobile nursing services and community health services targeted especially for certain conditions, for example maternity, family planning and sexual

health services, mental health services and dentistry, or those using particular therapies such as physiotherapy, chiropractic and osteopathy services (New Zealand Ministry of Health 2003).

Primary Health Organisations (PHOs) are:

> . . . the local structures for delivering and coordinating primary health care services [and they] bring together doctors, nurses and other health professionals (such as Māori health workers, health promotion workers, dieticians, pharmacists, physiotherapists, psychologists and midwives) in the community to serve the needs of their enrolled populations (New Zealand Ministry of Health 2003).

There are 81 PHOs around New Zealand. The PHOs are not-for-profit organisations and they are funded by the government to provide services within the DHBs (see Fig 3.2).

The New Zealand healthcare system provides public and private healthcare services. Eligible persons are entitled to receive free public health and subsidised medicines. Disabled people are eligible to receive various community-based services. The Ministry of Health has funding known as the **Special High Cost Treatment Pool**, available for people needing specialised one-off (not ongoing) treatment. The DHB applies to the government for this funding on behalf of the person needing the treatment (New Zealand Ministry of Health 2003).

The New Zealand **Accident Compensation Corporation (ACC)**, or Te Kaporeihana Awhina Hunga Whara, administers the compulsory **accident compensation scheme**. Under this scheme, New Zealand citizens, residents and temporary visitors to New Zealand are covered for personal injury. The scheme operates to cover the costs involved for the compensation and care of people who have been injured. People who have sustained injuries do not have the right to sue for personal injury (Accident Compensation Corporation 2007).

New Zealanders can choose to purchase private health insurance for a fee or '**premium**' directly from a private health insurance company, also known as a **private health fund**. Individuals or families can have private health insurance policies. This means that they can use private health services, and can avoid public hospital waiting lists for elective surgery by going to a private hospital and have a choice of which doctors to engage in private hospitals. The patient then receives a refund for hospital or other non-hospital health services. Depending on the level of insurance, also called '**cover**', there may be '**out-of-pocket' expenses** or '**gaps**' if the practitioner or service charges the patient more than the insurance company will refund (i.e. more than the **scheduled fee**).

Rights and responsibilities for New Zealand healthcare consumers

Under the **Health and Disability Commissioner Act**, the **Code of Health and Disability Services Consumers' Rights** became law on 1 July 1996 (and was reviewed in 1999 and reviewed and amended in 2004).

The **Health and Disability Commission (HDC)** asserts that, under the Act, health professionals must take 'reasonable actions in the circumstances to give effect to the rights, and comply with the duties in the Code' (Health and Disability Commission undated-a).

FIGURE 3.2 Overview of the New Zealand health and disability system and services

New Zealand Ministry of Health

Policy
Regulation
Funding
Monitoring

Directorates including the Māori Health Directorate

District Health Boards (DHBs) $n = 21$

Funding services in district
Provision of services in district

Primary Health Organisations (PHOs) $n = 81$

Delivery and coordination of healthcare services in local area

↓

Health services

Public
(includes the Special High Cost Treatment Pool)

Levels/degrees
Primary care—community
Secondary care—hospitals
Tertiary care—specialised doctors

Needs-based
Acute (e.g. medical-surgical, specialised)
Subacute (e.g. rehabilitation, palliative, interim)
Residential (e.g. aged, disability)
Community (e.g. aged care in home)

Health focus
Maternity
Mental health
Disability
Aged
Palliative
Indigenous
Chronic health conditions (e.g. diabetes)
And others

Private
Natural therapies (some private health insurance companies provide refunds)

The Code applies to any person or organisation who provides health services under the public health system, and to all persons and services who provide any form of care for people with disabilities (and is not restricted to the public system). All registered health professionals, as well as those who provide 'alternative', complementary, natural or holistic medicine services, are required to abide by the Code (Health and Disability Commission undated-a). The Code is summarised in Table 3.2.

TABLE 3.2 Summary of the Code of Health and Disability Services Consumers' Rights in New Zealand

Consumers of health and disability services have the following rights:	
Right 1:	Right to be treated with respect
Right 2:	Right to freedom from discrimination, coercion, harassment and exploitation
Right 3:	Right to dignity and independence
Right 4:	Right to services of an appropriate standard
Right 5:	Right to effective communication
Right 6:	Right to be fully informed
Right 7:	Right to make an informed choice and give informed consent
Right 8:	Right to support
Right 9:	Rights in respect of teaching or research
Right 10:	Right to complain

Source: Health and Disability Commission undated-b.

Models of healthcare in Australia and New Zealand

In both Australia and New Zealand, the biomedical approach to health guides the practice of **Western medicine** and is the dominant model of healthcare, although other (natural therapy) approaches are increasingly popular.

The Western biomedical approach to health

Within the Western **biomedical model** of health, science is considered to be an important basis for understanding health and treatment. Illness or disease is viewed as a problem that requires treatment—usually drugs or surgery, for example. The primary, secondary and tertiary levels of healthcare originate from the biomedical model of healthcare, with a medical practitioner (doctor) often the main provider of care. It is important to note that the healthcare systems in Western countries also address public health, preventative medicine and health promotion. **Primary healthcare (PHC)** is considered to be particularly important.

Primary healthcare

Primary healthcare is a philosophy that guides a particular approach to healthcare, and aims to overcome inequities in healthcare. PHC was first described in the *Declaration of Alma Ata* (at a conference of the World Health Organization (WHO) and UNICEF) in 1978. The Australian Primary Health Care Research Institute (APHCRI) defines PHC as:

> Socially appropriate, universally accessible, scientifically sound first level care provided by a suitably trained workforce supported by integrated referral systems and in a way that gives priority to those most in need, maximises community and individual self-reliance and participation and involves collaboration with other sectors. It includes health promotion, illness prevention, care of the sick, advocacy and community development (Sibthorpe et al 2005 p S52).

Other approaches to health

Other approaches to health are popular in Australia and New Zealand. These approaches are known by many terms, including **alternative**, **complementary**, **natural**, **holistic** or **traditional medicine/therapies**, or **complementary and alternative medicine (CAM)**. The philosophies, theories and practices of these approaches differ from the Western biomedical approach, and are based on understandings of nature and a fundamental belief in the importance of an holistic approach, which includes the physical, mental, emotional, spiritual, social and environmental aspects of the human person and health (Cuthbertson 2008 p 103, Fontaine 2005 pp 3–45, Birks & Chapman 2009 Ch 35).

Many people consult chiropractors, osteopaths, Chinese medicine practitioners, naturopaths, homeopaths and other natural therapy practitioners for complementary healthcare (in addition to Western medical care) or alternative healthcare (instead of Western medical care). In both Australia and New Zealand, many nurses have an interest in natural therapies (McCabe 2001 pp 7–21), and there are many resources for the integration of natural therapies into nursing practice (Cuthbertson 2008 pp 116–17, Fontaine 2005 pp 18–22, Birks & Chapman 2009 Ch 35). In New Zealand, national standards for traditional Māori healing were developed and published in 1999. These emphasised the role of ronga Māori (herbal medicine) within the health sector (Māori Health undated-d).

? QUESTION FOR REFLECTION

What is the dominant model of healthcare in your country, and how popular is it compared with the traditional medicine of your culture?

Healthcare services in Australia and New Zealand

Healthcare services in Australia and New Zealand are funded, managed and delivered in various ways. Various levels of government and organisations provide healthcare services (see Figs 3.1 and 3.2 above).

Many terms are used to describe healthcare, healthcare facilities and services, and the type of care provided.

Levels of care: primary, secondary and tertiary care

The levels of healthcare are referred to as primary, secondary and tertiary care. **Primary care** refers to the services provided to people in their communities. It is important to note that primary care is not a philosophy (like 'primary healthcare'). This can be confusing, as sometimes the terms are used interchangeably. Primary care is a way of describing a person's first point of contact with or entry to the healthcare system. For example, a local doctor (also known as a general practitioner or GP) provides primary care to people. Other health professionals, including dentists, physiotherapists, chiropractors, dieticians and nurses, also provide primary care.

Secondary care refers to the healthcare provided by hospitals. A number of health professionals provide care to hospitalised people, including doctors, nurses, pharmacists, psychologists and physiotherapists. Allied health professionals, including occupational therapists, dieticians and social workers, are also employed by hospitals in Australia and New Zealand.

Tertiary care means the specialised care provided typically by specialist medical practitioners. This could include care from a surgeon (which could be provided in a hospital that has the ability to deliver tertiary healthcare).

Needs and locations: acute, subacute, residential and community care

The degree of healthcare needs experienced by the person (e.g. **acute care** or **subacute care**), and sometimes the location where the care is delivered (e.g. **community care** or **residential care**), are used to broadly classify the type of care or describe the healthcare service (see Table 3.3).

Health focus

Some services are described according to their health focus. These include maternity, mental health, aged care and palliative care services. Some services are condition or disease specific, such as those that address diabetes, arthritis, asthma and depression. These services could be involved in research, education, health promotion, support, referral or treatment for the condition or disease.

Public and private services

The health services could be further described according to the type of ownership and business model. They could be public, private, affiliated with church groups or charities, **not-for-profit**, or combinations of these. In Australia and New Zealand, not-for-profit means that the money made by the organisation is returned to the organisation. For example, a private not-for-profit hospital (which is most likely affiliated with a religious group) could use its profit to purchase equipment or renovate a ward. In a private hospital that is operated as a business, the profit is retained by the owner(s) of the business. In New Zealand, the PHOs are not-for-profit.

Some examples of the types of facilities that provide healthcare services are listed in Table 3.3. There are many more services and facilities that you will discover while studying and working in Australia and New Zealand.

?

QUESTION FOR REFLECTION

What types of healthcare facilities are available in your country and how do these compare to those available in Australia and New Zealand?

Specialised health services

Indigenous health in Australia and New Zealand

In both Australia and New Zealand, there are Indigenous populations (**Aboriginal** and **Torres Strait Islanders** in Australia and **Māori** in New Zealand) whose health status is generally much worse than the rest of the population. Various government strategies, policies and programs exist, with the aim of overcoming the social, economic, educational and health disadvantages experienced by Indigenous people in both countries. Healthcare services and professionals are also involved in Indigenous health initiatives.

In Australia, Aboriginal and Torres Strait Islander people experience:

> . . . lower incomes than the non-Indigenous population, higher rates of unemployment, poorer educational outcomes and lower rates of home ownership—all of which can

TABLE 3.3 Healthcare facilities and services

Type of service/definition	Examples of facilities	Care
Acute Provides care for acute health needs. They: • are public *or* private • could be not-for-profit • could be religious/charity	General hospital (medical/surgical)	Acute medical and surgical care
	Specialised hospitals: • children's hospital • women's hospital • cancer centre • eye and ear hospital • dental hospital	Acute medical and surgical care to meet specialised needs
Subacute Provides care for non-acute health needs. They: • are public *or* private • could be not-for-profit • could be religious/charity	Rehabilitation hospital (or a rehabilitation unit/ward within a general hospital)	Rehabilitation care to assist optimal function
	Interim care (or an interim care unit/ward within a general hospital)	Care for older people who are waiting for residential care placement (often follows an acute admission)
	Palliative care or hospice (or a palliative care unit/ward within a general hospital)	Care for people who are dying
Residential Provides permanent care for people who live in the facility. They: • are public *or* private • could be not-for-profit • could be religious/charity	Aged care—low-level care: • supported residential service (SRS) or hostel	Residential care for older people who need assistance with personal care (person must have some functional independence)
	Aged care—high-level care: • nursing home	Residential care for older people who need nursing care (person could be fully dependent)
	Disabled: • community residential unit (CRU)	Residential care in a group home for people with physical and/or intellectual disabilities
	Mental health: • community residential unit (CRU)	Residential care in a group home for people with psychiatric/mental health needs
Community Provided in the community via an organisation or private practitioner. They: • are public *or* private • could be not-for-profit • could be religious/charity	Maternal and child health services	Care for babies/children and mothers/families
	Community aged care	Care for older people in the community—could include meal delivery, home help, transport, personal care
	Visiting or mobile nursing services	Community nursing care delivered in the person's home (e.g. wound, medication or diabetes management)

TABLE 3.3 Healthcare facilities and services—*cont'd*

Type of service/definition	Examples of facilities	Care
Community	'Hospital in the home' services	Acute care managed by the hospital and delivered to people in their homes (e.g. chemotherapy). Avoids acute hospital admission
	Domestic assistance	Home cleaning for people in need
	Meal delivery service	Meals delivered to people in need in their homes

impact upon a person's health and wellbeing (Australian Institute of Health and Welfare 2006).

In 1994, the Australian Government established the Office for Aboriginal and Torres Strait Islander Health (OATSIH) and its long-term strategy is:

> . . . to improve the access of Aboriginal and Torres Strait Islander peoples to comprehensive primary health care services. The aim is to provide coordinated clinical care, population health and health promotion activities to facilitate illness prevention, early intervention and effective disease management (Office for Aboriginal and Torres Strait Islander Health 2006).

In addition, the National Aboriginal and Torres Strait Islander Health Council provides advice to the Minister for Health and Ageing on government policy and program delivery relating to the health of Indigenous Australians (National Aboriginal and Torres Strait Islander Health Council 2006).

The New South Wales (NSW) state health department has prepared a document for health professionals to assist them in using appropriate language when communicating with Indigenous Australians. It is recommended that you obtain a copy of this publication, listed in 'Recommended reading' (New South Wales Health 2004).

'As a population group, Māori have on average the poorest health status of any ethnic group in New Zealand' (Māori Health undated-a). The Māori Health Directorate is a part of the New Zealand Ministry of Health and its roles are:

> . . . to provide policy advice on the overall strategy for achieving the government's objective for health, which is to reduce inequalities in health status for Māori and improve Māori health and disability status . . . and to develop relationships with the key organisations and agencies that contribute to a health and disability sector with a view to improving Māori health and disability status, and facilitating leadership within the Māori health sector (Māori Health Directorate undated).

The Māori Health Strategy (He Korowai Oranga) is incorporated in the New Zealand Health Strategy and is based on three principles: 'Partnership, Participation and Protection [which] are clearly articulated in line with Māori expectations of their relationship with the Crown in the health and disability sector' (Māori Health undated-b).

Chapter 6 addresses issues related to Māori health, and provides examples of culturally appropriate care and examples of Māori terminology.

Blood services

The Australian Red Cross Blood Service and the New Zealand Blood Service are the national organisations that coordinate the collection and distribution of blood and blood products for transfusion in Australia and New Zealand respectively. In both countries, blood donation is voluntary and unpaid.

Rural and remote area services in Australia

Due to the limited health resources available for people living in some rural and remote areas of Australia, there have been a number of government initiatives—referred to collectively as rural health services—to improve the availability of and access to healthcare for these communities (Australian Government Department of Health and Ageing 2006).

In Australia, there are very large areas of land that are sparsely populated. Access to healthcare in these remote areas can be extremely difficult, as there are few facilities and few health professionals. Unique services, such as the Royal Flying Doctor Service (RFDS), are an important part of remote area healthcare in Australia. RFDS is a 'not-for-profit charitable service providing aeromedical emergency and primary healthcare services together with communication and education assistance to people who live, work and travel in regional and remote Australia' (Royal Flying Doctor Service 2006).

Health professionals in Australia and New Zealand

In Australia and New Zealand, there are many health professionals who provide healthcare. In many cases, the education and practice of health professionals is regulated.

It is important for you to be aware of the terms related to other health professionals, as well as the care they provide. While some of the health professionals will be the same in your country, others will be different.

Registration of health professionals

In Australia and New Zealand, it is law that certain health professionals—including some natural health professionals—be **registered** with a **professional board** (sometimes called a statutory authority or regulatory authority) before practising their professions (including doctors, nurses, pharmacists, dentists and chiropractors), but a number are not. The education and training of registered health professionals is regulated. This means that approved institutions (such as a university) must provide accredited courses (such as a Bachelor of Nursing), in order to meet the criteria for registration with the professional board or regulatory authority (such as the Nurses Board of Victoria or the Nursing Council of New Zealand). Accreditation for courses and approval for institutions that provide the courses are given by the regulatory authority.

In New Zealand, there is a single national law called the **Health Practitioners Competence Assurance Act (HPCAA)** 2003, which regulates the practice of all registered health professions (New Zealand Ministry of Health 2006), including chiropractors, dentists, dieticians, medical laboratory technologists and scientists, medical practitioners, medical radiation technologists, midwives, nurses, occupational therapists, optometrists, osteopaths, pharmacists, physiotherapists, podiatrists and psychologists (Nursing Council of New Zealand 2008). There are separate national registration authorities for many of the different health professions, such as the Nursing Council of New Zealand.

In Australia, the individual state and territory laws govern the education and registration of many health professionals, with separate boards existing in each state and territory for many of the registered professions. For example, the Nurses Board of Victoria and the Nurses and Midwives Board of New South Wales regulate nursing practice only in their respective states. There are some differences between the states and territories, regarding which professionals must be registered.

A new national system has been proposed by the Council of Australian Governments (COAG) and is due to be implemented by July 2010 (Council of Australian Governments 2008b). A national law will be introduced to govern the education and registration of health professionals, and national boards will be established for each of the nine health professionals initially affected: medical practitioners (doctors), nurses and midwives, pharmacists, physiotherapists, psychologists, osteopaths, chiropractors, optometrists and dentists (including dental hygienists, dental prosthetists and dental therapists) (Council of Australian Governments 2008a).

Terminology associated with health professionals

In your study and practice you will need to be familiar with many terms associated with health professionals. The following list includes some of them.

Medical

- **Medical practitioner/doctor**: general terms; have the same meaning to describe a professional who provides medical care or 'practises medicine' (this could include surgery).
- **Consultant/specialist**: senior doctor who has specialised training in a particular field; usually have a private practice (in the community) and also work in hospitals (e.g. vascular surgeon, renal physician, cardiologist, urologist, psychiatrist).
- **Registrar**: doctor with more than 1 or 2 years' experience, working in the hospital system (could be training in a specialty area) (e.g. neurology registrar, orthopaedic registrar).
- **Resident**: junior doctor with 1 or 2 years' experience, working in the hospital system.
- **Intern**: graduate doctor in first year of practice, working in the hospital system. (Note: In some states of the United States of America (USA), an intern is the term for a registrar, and an internist is a consultant who specialises in internal medicine.)
- **General practitioner (GP)**: a doctor who provides primary care from a community-based practice (these doctors are generally not hospital employees in Australia or New Zealand).

Nursing (see Ch 4)

- **Registered nurse (RN)** or **registered nurse (Division 1) (RN Div 1)**: general nurse, able to practise in a broad range of areas.

- **Enrolled nurse (EN)/registered nurse (Division 2) (RN Div 2)**: second-level nurse whose practice is generally supervised by a registered nurse or registered nurse (Div 1).
- **Mental health nurse/psychiatric nurse**: registered nurse or registered nurse (Div 1) with postgraduate qualifications in mental health nursing *or* mental health nurse whose practice is limited to mental health nursing.
- **Midwife**: registered nurse or registered nurse (Div 1) with postgraduate qualifications in midwifery *or* midwife whose practice is limited to midwifery.
- **Mothercraft nurse**: formerly a person who had a qualification in basic care of the newborn and assisted midwives in postnatal care. Their practice was limited to mothercraft nursing only.

Paramedics

- **Paramedic**: a professional trained to deliver first aid and emergency care via a mobile service (where the vehicle is called an ambulance).
- **MICA paramedic**: an ambulance officer who is trained in advanced skills and able to work in the mobile intensive care ambulance (MICA) service. (MICA vehicles carry intensive care equipment and MICA paramedics can intubate patients who require ventilation.)

Dental

- **Dentist**: a specialist who provides dental care (pertaining to the teeth and mouth).
- **Dental hygienist/therapist**: provides auxiliary dental care, working with and under the general supervision of a dentist. Dental hygienists/therapists are the primary care providers of school dental healthcare.
- **Dental prosthetist**: makes dental prosthetics (dentures).

Allied health

- **Dietician**: assesses and advises about nutritional needs, including special diets.
- **Nuclear medicine technologist**: administers radiation for diagnostic or therapeutic use.
- **Occupational therapist (OT)**: specialises in the assessment of functional ability and provides aids for optimal independence (related to personal care, domestic or occupational activities).
- **Optometrist**: assesses eye health and prescribes aids for vision.
- **Pharmacist**: supplies, dispenses and advises on the use of medicines in hospital settings and community pharmacies ('chemist shops').
- **Physiotherapist**: specialises in the assessment and treatment of the musculoskeletal system. The aim of physiotherapy is to achieve optimal mobility.
- **Psychologist**: specialises in human behaviour; provides assessments of emotional and mental health, as well as other aspects of behaviour, and provides counselling and advice.
- **Podiatrist**: assesses and treats the feet. A podiatrist is not a specialist doctor/medical practitioner in Australia or New Zealand.
- **Radiographer**: operates radiological equipment (e.g. X-ray machines).
- **Social worker**: assists people with adaptation to social circumstances; also provides individual, family or group counselling.

- **Speech pathologist** (formerly known as a speech therapist): assesses and assists difficulties with communication, speech, swallowing and feeding.

Indigenous health workers

- **Aboriginal and Torres Strait Islander health worker/Aboriginal health worker**: acts as liaison between Indigenous Australians and health professionals, and also provides support, information and healthcare to Indigenous people.
- **Māori health worker**: provides advocacy, support, information and education to Māori people. Some Māori health workers are also registered nurses.

Natural therapists (natural/alternative/complementary medicine practitioners)

- **Chinese medicine practitioner**: a specialist in the Traditional Chinese Medicine (TCM) system that includes the use of herbs, massage and acupuncture.
- **Chiropractor**: a specialist in the chiropractic system of healthcare, which focuses on the assessment and adjustment of the neuromusculoskeletal system through manipulation, massage, diet and exercise.
- **Homeopath**: a specialist in homeopathy, which is a complex system based on the belief that 'like cures like', where extremely dilute remedies of a substance which could cause a condition is used to treat that same condition. Homeopathy is sometimes classified as a form of energy-based medicine.
- **Masseur/massage therapist**: uses massage for relaxation and therapeutic purposes.
- **Naturopath**: a specialist in Western alternative medicine (naturopathy), which includes massage, herbal medicine, diet and, in cases where the practitioner has additional education, may incorporate homeopathy or other natural modalities.
- **Nurse practitioner**: a registered nurse who is authorised (by a nursing regulatory authority) to practise autonomously in an advanced clinical role, in a particular specialty area of practice.
- **Osteopath**: a specialist in osteopathy, which is based on the belief that musculoskeletal system problems could be a reflection of other problems in the body, and uses techniques including manipulation, diet and exercise to improve health.
- **Reflexologist**: uses specialised massage techniques to stimulate reflex areas (that reflect certain other organs or parts) in the feet (or hands). Reflexology is based on specific understandings of energy flow, which are similar to the meridians associated with acupuncture.
- **Traditional Aboriginal medicine (bush medicine) healer**: practises traditional healing methods that include spiritual healing by special healers (like shamans) to remove evil spirits, as well as ceremonies and rituals to improve health and herbal medicine (Devanesen 2000).
- **Traditional Māori healer**: practises traditional healing that is 'based on a wellness or holistic health model' (Māori Health undated-c), and uses methods including massage, herbs and prayer. Spirituality is considered to be particularly important (Māori Health undated-d).

Non-professionals

- **Assistant in nursing (AIN) (Aus)**: see personal care attendant.
- **Carer**: see personal care attendant.

- **Domestic staff/cleaner**: provides cleaning services in healthcare services.
- **Healthcare assistant (NZ)**: see personal care attendant.
- **Kitchen staff/cook**: prepares meals (and in health facilities such as hospitals or nursing homes could be required to liaise with dieticians and/or registered nurses to meet special diet needs for patients).
- **Medical receptionist**: does administrative work and manages the appointments in a medical centre (e.g. a GP practice).
- **Orderly**: assists with patient transport around the hospital by moving trolleys or wheelchairs.
- **Personal care attendant (PCA) (Aus)**—also referred to as **carer/personal carer/personal care worker (PCW) (Aus)/assistant in nursing (AIN) (Aus)/ healthcare assistant (NZ)/support care worker (NZ)**: provides basic assistance with personal care (i.e. mobility, hygiene, grooming, feeding and toileting) and is usually employed to assist people in their homes, or by residential disability facilities or residential aged care facilities. (In nursing homes, the PCA must be supervised by a registered nurse (Div 1) or registered nurse.)
- **Personal carer**: see personal care attendant.
- **Personal care worker (PCW) (Aus)**: see personal care attendant.
- **Support care worker (NZ)**: see personal care attendant.
- **Ward clerk**: does clerical or administrative work on a ward in a hospital setting.

?

QUESTION FOR REFLECTION

Do the same types of health professionals practise in your country?

CHAPTER HIGHLIGHTS

- The Australian and New Zealand healthcare systems are considered to be advanced and of a high standard.
- Democratically elected governments are ultimately responsible for healthcare.
- In Australia, the federal, state/territory and local governments share the responsibility for healthcare services.
- In New Zealand, the Ministry of Health, District Health Boards and Primary Care Organisations share the responsibility for healthcare services.
- In Australia and New Zealand, there are public and private healthcare systems.
- In Australia, there are currently separate state and territory charters of patients' rights (for public hospitals) and a national private health system charter.
- In New Zealand, the HDC Code of Health and Disability Services Consumers' Rights outlines the rights of health and disability service users, which health professionals are required by law to uphold.
- While the Western biomedical approach is the dominant model of health, natural therapies—also known as complementary and alternative medicine—are increasingly popular.
- Healthcare services can be classified according to:
  —the level of care provided (primary, secondary or tertiary)

—health needs or location (acute, subacute, residential, community), and
—health focus (e.g. maternity, mental health, aged care, palliative care).

- In Australia, there are various government strategies, policies and programs aimed at addressing the health inequities experienced by Indigenous Australians (Aboriginal and Torres Strait Islanders).
- In New Zealand, there are various government strategies, policies and programs aimed at addressing the health inequities experienced by Indigenous New Zealanders (Māori).
- In Australia and New Zealand, specialised healthcare services exist to meet the needs of the population.
- In Australia and New Zealand, there are laws governing the education, registration and practice of many health professionals, including nurses. In both countries, nurses must be registered with the relevant nursing regulatory authority in order to practise.
- Various health professionals practise in Australian and New Zealand healthcare settings.

Self-test questions

Plain numbered questions are for all readers; 'a' questions are for readers in Australia; 'b' questions are for readers in New Zealand.

1a. On a map of Australia, identify the states and territories and their capital cities.

1b. On a map of New Zealand, identify the islands and major cities.

2a. What are the responsibilities of the Commonwealth, state/territory and local government sectors within the Australian healthcare system?

2b. What are the responsibilities of the Crown, the District Health Boards and the Primary Care Organisations within the New Zealand health and disability system?

3a. Describe the types of healthcare services available in Australia.

3b. Describe the types of healthcare services available in New Zealand.

4a. Read the relevant public hospital charter of patients' rights and responsibilities for your state or territory from the following websites:

Australian Capital Territory: www.health.act.gov.au/c/health?a=sendfile&ft=p&fid=1190160455&sid=

New South Wales: www.health.nsw.gov.au/health-public-affairs/you/charter.html

Northern Territory: www.nt.gov.au/omb_hcscc/hcscc/pdf/Code.pdf

Queensland: www.health.qld.gov.au/qhppc/documents/QHPPCbrochure.pdf

South Australia: www.safetyandquality.sa.gov.au/Default.aspx?tabid=68

Tasmania: www.dhhs.tas.gov.au/services/view.php?id=602

Victoria: www.health.vic.gov.au/patientcharter/patient.htm

Western Australia: www.health.wa.gov.au/services/downloads/Hospital_Charter-Brochure.pdf

List some implications of the charter for your nursing practice in Australia (provide clinical-based examples).

4b. Read the Code of Health and Disability Services Consumers' Rights Regulation 1996 from the following website: www.hdc.org.nz/theact/theact-thecodedetail. List some implications of the code for your nursing practice in New Zealand (provide clinical-based examples).

5. List some differences between the Western biomedical model of health and alternative/complementary/holistic/natural medicine therapies.

6. Read and summarise a recent journal article about natural therapies in nursing using the 'Article summary sheet' (R1) on the CD Part 3—Reader resources.

7a. Read and summarise a recent journal article about the health of Indigenous Australians using the 'Article summary sheet' (R1) on the CD Part 3—Reader resources.

7b. Read and summarise a recent journal article about the health of Māori using the 'Article summary sheet' (R1) on the CD Part 3—Reader resources.

8. What is the name of the law that governs the practice of nurses where you are working or studying?

9. Explain the concept of registration for nurses and discuss why it is considered to be important.

10. Define the types of health professionals listed in this chapter.

11. Review the key terms and any other new vocabulary, terms and abbreviations from this chapter, and then update your 'Language list' (R2) on the CD Part 3—Reader resources.

12. Answer the 'Learning objectives' at the start of this chapter as if they were examination questions.

References

Accident Compensation Corporation 2007 About ACC. Online. Available www.acc.co.nz/about-acc/index.htm 20 Feb 2008

ACT Health 2007 ACT Health: your rights and responsibilities. Online. Available www.health.act.gov.au/c/health?a=sendfile&ft=p&fid=1190160455&sid= 28 Nov 2007

Australian Bureau of Statistics 2001 Australian social trends 2001. Online. Available www.abs.gov.au/AUSSTATS/abs@.nsf/7d12b0f6763c78caca257061001cc588/964f93de8bb5c425ca2570ec000bf8f8!OpenDocument 20 June 2007

Australian Bureau of Statistics 2008 Population clock. Online. Available www.abs.gov.au/Ausstats/ABS@.nsf/94713ad445ff1425ca25682000192af2/1647509ef7e25faaca2568a900154b63!OpenDocument 4 Mar 2008

Australian Government Department of Health and Ageing 2006 Rural health services. Online. Available www.health.gov.au/internet/wcms/publishing.nsf/Content/ruralhealth-services-index.htm 10 May 2007

Australian Government Department of Health and Ageing 2007 Private Patients' Hospital Charter. Online. Available www.health.gov.au/internet/wcms/publishing.nsf/Content/privatehealth-hospital-charter-contents.htm 28 Nov 2007

Australian Institute of Health and Welfare 2006 Indigenous Australians. Online. Available www.aihw.gov.au/indigenous/ 7 May 2007

Birks M, Chapman Y 2009 Complementary therapies in practice. In Crisp J, Taylor C (eds) Potter & Perry's fundamentals of nursing, 3rd edn. Elsevier, Sydney, Ch 35

Commonwealth Department of Health and Aged Care 2000 The Australian health care system: an outline. Online. Available www.health.gov.au/internet/wcms/publishing.nsf/Content/haf-ozhealth-index 7 May 2007

Council of Australian Governments 2008a Council of Australian Governments' Communique, 26 March 2008. Online. Available www.coag.gov.au/meetings/ 130407/ 12 May 2008

Council of Australian Governments 2008b Intergovernmental agreement for a national registration and accreditation scheme for the health professions. Online. Available www.coag.gov.au/meetings/260308/docs/iga_health_workforce.rtf / 12 May 2008

Cuthbertson L 2008 Complementary and alternative therapies. In: Brown D, Edwards H (eds) Lewis's medical–surgical nursing: assessment and management of clinical problems, 2nd edn. Elsevier, Sydney, pp 103–20. Adapted from Shaw V 2008 Complementary and alternative therapies. In: Brown D, Edwards H (eds) Lewis's medical–surgical nursing: assessment and management of clinical problems, 2nd edn. Elsevier, Sydney, pp 103–20

Department of Health and Human Services Tasmania 2005 Your rights and responsibilities: patient information. Online. Available www.dhhs.tas.gov.au/services/view.php?id=602 28 Nov 2007

Department of Health South Australia 2005 Your rights and responsibilities. A charter for South Australian public health system consumers. Online. Available www.safetyandquality.sa.gov.au/Default.aspx?tabid=68 28 Nov 2007

Department of Health Western Australia 2004 The Western Australian public patient hospital charter. Online. Available www.health.wa.gov.au/services/downloads/Hospital_Charter-Brochure.pdf 28 Nov 2007

Department of Human Services Victoria 2007 Public hospital patient charter. Online. Available www.health.vic.gov.au/patientcharter/patient.htm 28 Nov 2007

Devanesen D 2000 Traditional Aboriginal medicine practice in the Northern Territory. Paper presented at the International Symposium of traditional medicine: better science, policy and services for health development, 11–13 September 2000, Awaji Island, Japan. Online. Available www.nt.gov.au/health/comm_health/abhealth_strategy/Traditional%20Aboriginal%20Medicine%20-%20Japan%20Paper.pdf 10 June 2007

Fontaine KL 2005 Complementary and alternative medicine for nursing practice, 2nd edn. Pearson, Upper Saddle River, New Jersey

Health and Community Services Complaints Commission Northern Territory undated Code of health and community responsibilities. Online. Available www.nt.gov.au/omb_hcscc/hcscc/pdf/Code.pdf 28 Nov 2007

Health and Disability Commission undated-a The code of health and disability services consumers' rights. Online. Available www.hdc.org.nz/theact/theact-thecode 28 Nov 2007

Health and Disability Commission undated-b The HDC Code of Health and Disability Services Consumers' Rights Regulation 1996. Online. Available www.hdc.org.nz/theact/theact-thecodedetail 28 Nov 2007

Māori Health undated-a About Māori health. Online. Available www.maorihealth.govt.nz/moh.nsf/menuma/About+Maori+Health 10 May 2007

Māori Health undated-b Addressing Māori health. Online. Available www.maorihealth.govt.nz/moh.nsf/pagesma/304?Open 10 May 2007

Māori Health undated-c Māori health models. Online. Available www.maorihealth.govt.nz/moh.nsf/pagesma/196 10 May 2007

Māori Health undated-d Traditional Māori healing. Online. Available www.maorihealth.govt.nz/moh.nsf/pagesma/194 10 May 2007

Māori Health Directorate undated Welcome to Te Kete Hanuora: the Māori Health Directorate. Online. Available www.moh.govt.nz/moh.nsf/pagesma/321 10 May 2007

McCabe P 2001 Nursing and complementary therapies: a natural partnership. In: McCabe P (ed) Complementary therapies in nursing and midwifery: from vision to practice. Ausmed, Ascot Vale, Victoria, pp 7–22

National Aboriginal and Torres Strait Islander Health Council 2006 National Aboriginal and Torres Strait Islander Health Council. Online. Available www.health.gov.au/internet/wcms/publishing.nsf/Content/health-oatsih-healthcouncil 7 May 2007

New South Wales Health 2005 You and your health service: patient charter. Online. Available www.health.nsw.gov.au/health-public-affairs/you/charter.html 28 Nov 2007

Newton PW 2001 Australia state of the environment: human settlements theme report. Online. Available www.environment.gov.au/soe/2001/settlements/settlements01.html 20 June 2007

New Zealand Ministry of Health 2003 The New Zealand health and disability system 2003. Online. Available www.moh.govt.nz/healthsystem 7 May 2007
New Zealand Ministry of Health 2006 Health Practitioners Competence Assurance Act 2003. Online. Available www.moh.govt.nz/hpca 12 May 2007
Nursing Council of New Zealand 2008 Health Practitioners Competence Assurance Act 2003. Online. Available www.nursingcouncil.org.nz/hpca.html 13 May 2008
Office for Aboriginal and Torres Strait Islander Health 2006 About OATSIH. Online. Available www.health.gov.au/internet/wcms/publishing.nsf/Content/health-oatsih-about 7 May 2007
Queensland Health 2007 Queensland Health public patients' charter. Online. Available www.health.qld.gov.au/qhppc/documents/QHPPCbrochure.pdf 28 Nov 2007
Royal Flying Doctor Service 2006 Royal Flying Doctor Service of Australia. Online. Available www.flyingdoctor.net/who.htm 17 May 2007
Sibthorpe BM, Glasgow NJ, Wells RW 2005 Questioning the sustainability of primary health care innovation. Medical Journal of Australia 183(10):S52–S53 Online. Available www.mja.com.au/public/issues/183_10_211105/sib10638_fm.html 13 May 2008
Statistics New Zealand 2006a 2006 Census of population and dwellings. Online. Available www.stats.govt.nz/NR/rdonlyres/ C2D66480-191C-4E9A-99A0-D64813DF2797/0/FinalCountTablesRCandTA1.xls 7 May 2007
Statistics New Zealand 2006d Quick stats about Māori. Online. Available www.stats.govt.nz/NR/rdonlyres/095030F8-BD62-4745-836D-0EF185619C37/0/2006censusquickstatsaboutmaorirevised.pdf 20 June 2007
Statistics New Zealand 2006e Quick stats about culture and identity. Online. Available www.stats.govt.nz/NR/rdonlyres/5F1F873C-5D36-4E54-9405-34503A2C0AF6/0/quickstatsaboutcultureandidentity.pdf 20 June 2007
Statistics New Zealand 2008 Population clock. Online. Available www.stats.govt.nz/populationclock.htm 12 May 2008

Recommended reading

New South Wales Health 2004 Communicating positively: a guide to appropriate Aboriginal terminology. Online. Available www.health.nsw.gov.au/pubs/2004/pdf/ab_terminology.pdf 5 Mar 2008

CHAPTER 4

Nursing in Australia and New Zealand

'There are many regulations and laws about nursing . . . it is very strict. I think this makes it safer for the patient.'

Mala, Sri Lanka

CHAPTER OUTLINE

LEARNING OBJECTIVES

1. Identify the Australian or New Zealand context for nursing.
2. Discuss the Australian or New Zealand regulatory frameworks for nursing.
3. Describe the type of nurses practising in Australia or New Zealand.
4. Discuss nursing education in Australia or New Zealand.

5. Describe the roles of the key nursing regulatory and professional bodies in Australia or New Zealand.
6. Identify key resources for nurses in Australia or New Zealand.

Key terms (are in bold in the text)

academics
accredited
Australian Nursing and Midwifery Council (ANMC)
Australian Nursing Federation (ANF)
Bachelor of Nursing (BN)
clinical placement
clinicians
College of Nurses Aotearoa New Zealand (CNA–NZ)
consultants
educators
enrolled nurse (EN)
leaders
managers
New Zealand Nurses Organisation (NZNO)
nurse assistant
nurse–patient ratio
nurse practitioners
nurse practitioner with prescribing rights
Nursing Council of New Zealand
nursing regulatory authority
nursing specialty areas
patient dependency system
practising certificate
registered nurse (RN)
registered nurse Divison 1 (RN Div 1)
registered nurse Divison 2 (RN Div 2)
researchers
Royal College of Nursing Australia (RCNA)
statutory nursing authority

To study and practise nursing in Australia or New Zealand, you need to be familiar with the contexts where nurses practise, nursing education, the types of nurses who practise in these countries and the roles they fulfil. It is essential to have a sound understanding of the regulation of nursing in both countries. In addition, understanding the roles and functions of the various nursing organisations that exist in Australia and New Zealand is important for all nursing students and nurses.

Nursing in Australia and New Zealand

Nurses in Australia and New Zealand are generally well respected and trusted health professionals. Nurses work in a range of settings and undertake various roles in the healthcare systems. Nurses are required to undertake formal education courses, which are internationally recognised as being of a high standard. All nurses must register with a **nursing regulatory authority** before being allowed to practise. In both Australia and New Zealand, nursing care is considered to be of a very high standard and all nurses, including students, are expected to be competent professionals. (Nursing standards and competencies are addressed in detail in Ch 5.)

Contexts for nursing in Australia and New Zealand

Nurses in Australia and New Zealand work in a diverse range of settings. Nurses are employed in the public and private healthcare sectors, in hospitals, aged care facilities and community organisations, in government facilities (including correctional centres or gaols) and government departments, in private companies and in primary healthcare services. Nurses work in urban, rural and remote areas.

Roles of nurses in Australia and New Zealand

The types of roles undertaken by nurses are also diverse. In Australia and New Zealand, nurses work as **clinicians**, **educators**, **academics**, **researchers**, **managers**, **consultants** and **leaders** in healthcare. Some nurses are **nurse practitioners**.

The **Australian Nursing and Midwifery Council (ANMC)** and the **Nursing Council of New Zealand** have a shared understanding of the role of the nurse practitioner and describe the nurse practitioner as 'a registered nurse educated and authorised to function autonomously and collaboratively in an advanced and extended clinical role' (Australian Nursing and Midwifery Council 2006 p 1). The nurse practitioner has very advanced knowledge, skills and education (and holds at least a master's degree) in a speciality area of practice. Nurse practitioners may have prescribing rights.

Nurse practitioners must have the endorsement noted on their practising certificate, which is issued by the nursing regulatory authority, or they must have a separate registration as a nurse practitioner. The term can *only* be used by those nurses who are endorsed or registered by a nursing regulatory authority as nurse practitioners and *must not* be used to describe a nurse who is practising as a clinical nurse.

Nursing workloads in Australia and New Zealand

It is generally considered that working conditions, and particularly nurses' workloads, in Australia and New Zealand are better than in many other countries. Workloads vary depending on the setting. In hospital settings, the number of nurses working in a ward or unit each shift is determined by either the **nurse–patient ratio** method, which is based on the type of ward, or predicted using a **patient dependency system**, which is based on patient acuity (or the needs of the patient).

In a study of nurse staffing in public and private hospitals in Australia, New Zealand and Thailand, it was found that both methods have a high correlation between the prediction and actualisation of nurses required—95.1% for the ratio method and 97.2% for the patient dependency method (Plummer 2005 p 21). In the Australian state of Victoria, nurse–patient ratios have been mandatory in the public health system since 2001, and this model has been proposed in New Zealand, but to date has not been implemented (O'Connor 2006).

Nursing in Australia

Regulation of nursing in Australia

Currently in Australia, the individual state and territory laws govern nursing in the respective states and territories.

In each state and territory, there is one **statutory nursing authority** or **nursing regulatory authority** responsible for governing the practice of nurses in that state or territory. (These are listed later in Table 4.3.) In some states and territories, there is a separate midwifery regulatory body.

Nurses must be registered with the relevant nursing regulatory authority and hold a current **practising certificate** (renewed annually). Nurses must be registered with the local nursing regulatory authority to practise in each state or territory. Under the Trans Tasman Mutual Recognition (TTMR) Act, there is a reciprocal registration agreement with New Zealand for all states and territories of Australia (Nursing Council of New Zealand 2008d).

Under the new national system proposed by the Council of Australian Governments (COAG) (due to commence in 2010), a national law will be introduced to govern the education and registration of health professionals, and national boards will be established for each of the nine health professionals initially affected, including nurses (Council of Australian Governments 2008a, 2008b).

QUESTION FOR REFLECTION

How is nursing regulated in your country and how does this compare to the regulation of nursing in Australia?

Types of nurses in Australia

In Australia, there are two levels of general nurse. While there are some differences in the categories or divisions of registration for nurses between the various state and territory nursing regulatory authorities, all have provision for the registration and/or enrolment of the two levels of nurse in Australia.

A **registered nurse (RN)**—also known as a **registered nurse Divison 1 (RN Div 1)** in Victoria—must have a **Bachelor of Nursing (BN)** or equivalent qualification. The second-level nurse is referred to as an **enrolled nurse (EN)**—also known as a **registered nurse Divison 2 (RN Div 2)** in Victoria—and must have an approved diploma or certificate for enrolment or registration with the local regulatory authority (Australian Nursing and Midwifery Council 2007j). (See Table 4.1.)

In the past, mental health nurses (known as psychiatric nurses) had a separate qualification and were able to practise only in the area of mental health, unless they had previously been registered nurses who then studied mental health nursing as a postgraduate specialty. Today, in most states and territories, registered nurses (RNs and RNs Div 1) who have a Bachelor of Nursing are qualified to practise in mental health nursing. Those who intend to work in this speciality usually undertake postgraduate study in mental health nursing.

In Australia, there are now two pathways for those who want to be midwives. As in the past, registered nurses (RNs and RNs Div 1) can undertake postgraduate studies in midwifery at university and then register as a midwife, and are referred to as a registered midwife (RM). Alternatively, those without nursing qualifications can now become midwives after undertaking a 3-year Bachelor of Midwifery (BM) at university (this is sometimes referred to as a direct entry program, because the student can enter the course directly, without having a nursing qualification). In some states and territories, midwifery is recognised as a separate discipline and there is a separate regulatory authority.

In Australia, unregistered carers are referred to as personal care attendants (PCAs), personal care workers (PCWs), personal carers or assistants in nursing (AINs), and are sometimes employed in the aged care or disability sectors and in home care situations. These workers are *not* nurses.

?

QUESTION FOR REFLECTION

What types of nurses are there in your country and how do they compare to the types of nurses in Australia?

Nursing education in Australia

In Australia, all teaching institutions (e.g. universities) who offer pre-registration nursing courses must be **accredited** by the nursing regulatory authority (in that state or territory). In addition, the course (which must include a clinical practice component, known as **clinical placement**) must be accredited by the nursing regulatory body. Registration as a nurse is only considered by the nursing regulatory authority for applicants who have successfully completed accredited courses at accredited intstitutions.

In general, students must complete an accredited Bachelor of Nursing course at an approved tertiary education institution (i.e. university) to apply for registration as a registered nurse or registered nurse (Div 1). Certificate or diploma courses for enrolled nurses or registered nurses (Div 2) must also be accredited by the local nursing regulatory authority and are usually provided by approved higher education institutes (institutes or colleges of technical and further education known as TAFE).

Pre-registration nursing education courses provide a combination of theoretical and practical education. Pre-registration nursing courses include subjects (sometimes called units) from the sciences (including anatomy, physiology, pathophysiology, pharmacology), the social sciences (including psychology and sociology), law and ethics, and more recently specific units about Indigenous issues and health. Core nursing subjects address the history, theory and practice of nursing, and the professional issues relevant to nurses. Many courses also offer some elective subjects, so students have the opportunity to study an area that is of interest to them.

Students are required to undertake a broad range of clinical placements in healthcare settings, such as hospitals, nursing homes, community health centres and mental health facilities. Clinical placement occurs throughout the course and students cannot be registered until the entire course has been successfully completed (unlike in some countries where a 2-year theoretical course is studied at college, followed by a 12-month clinical placement in a hospital). (Clinical placement is addressed in detail in Chs 12 and 13.)

There are many options for postgraduate nursing study. Nurses can study at the graduate certificate, graduate diploma, master's and doctoral or PhD level. There are a number of models for postgraduate nursing education in the clinical **nursing speciality areas**, including critical care, emergency, perioperative, neurosciences, plastics and vascular, anaesthetics and recovery, aged care, maternal and child health, mental health and midwifery. Courses are offered by universities, often in conjunction with a hospital that provides the clinical placement and clinical education. Some nurses also undertake non-nursing postgraduate studies in disciplines such as education and management.

Table 4.1 compares the education and practice of the types of nurses in Australia.

?

QUESTION FOR REFLECTION

How does nursing education in your country compare with nursing education in Australia?

TABLE 4.1 Nurses in Australia: classification, education and practice

Title	Educational qualification	Educational institute	Scope of practice	Notes
Registered nurse (RN) Registered nurse Division 1 (RN Div 1) (Victoria)	Bachelor of Nursing (or equivalent): 3 years	University (since 1980s) Hospital (prior to early 1990)	Diverse areas, including specialties with further postgraduate education	A **nurse practitioner** must be an RN/RN Div 1, with specific endorsement as a nurse practitioner
Enrolled nurse (EN) Registered nurse Division 2 (RN Div 2) (Victoria)	Diploma or certificate: 12–18 months Australian Capital Territory: Certificate IV in Health (Nursing) Northern Territory: Certificate IV in Community Services (EN) New South Wales: Certificate IV in Nursing (EN) Queensland: Diploma in Nursing South Australia: Diploma of Nursing (pre-enrolment) Tasmania: Certificate IV in Health (Nursing) Victoria: Certificate IV in Health (Nursing) Western Australia: Certificate IV in Enrolled Nursing *(Source: Australian Nursing and Midwifery Council 2007a, 2007b, 2007c, 2007d, 2007e, 2007f, 2007g, 2007h, 2007i and 2007l.)*	TAFE or TAFE/healthcare organisation—if undertaking a traineeship Hospital (prior to 1990s)	Restricted practice, second-level nurse Various areas (usually excluding acute specialties)	Formerly called state enrolled nurse (SEN) in Victoria
Registered midwife (RM)	Postgraduate—certificate/ diploma for RN/RN Div 1: 12 months minimum	University (since 1980s) or hospital (prior to early 1990)	Midwifery	Qualified to practise as RN/RN Div 1, RM
	Direct entry—Bachelor of Midwifery: 3 years	University (since early 2000s)		Qualified to practise as RM only

TABLE 4.1 Nurses in Australia: classification, education and practice—*cont'd*

Title	Educational qualification	Educational institute	Scope of practice	Notes
Mental health/psychiatric nurse (RN or RN Div 1) Former title: registered psychiatric nurse (RPN)	Bachelor of Nursing (or equivalent): 3 years	University	Mental health	Qualified to practise as RN/RN Div 1, which includes mental health nursing. Nurses who choose to specialise in this area usually undertake further studies
	Or in the past: Postgraduate certificate: 1 year	Psychiatric hospital		Qualified to practise as RN/RN Div 1 and RPN
	Psychiatric Nursing Certificate: 3 years	Psychiatric hospital		Practice restricted to mental health area only

Professional nursing organisations and resources in Australia

There are various nursing organisations and resources in Australia (see Tables 4.2 and 4.3). It is important to be familiar with the relevant nursing regulatory authority and with the professional bodies that represent nursing.

Nursing in New Zealand

Regulation of nursing in New Zealand

In New Zealand, there is single national law called the *Health Practitioners Competence Assurance Act* (HPCAA) 2003, which regulates the practice of all registered health professions (New Zealand Ministry of Health 2006).

The **Nursing Council of New Zealand** or Te Kaunihera Tapuhi o Aotearoa is the **statutory nursing authority** or **nursing regulatory authority** that governs the practice of nurses in New Zealand. 'The Council sets and monitors standards in the interests of the public and the profession . . . [and states that its] primary concern is public safety' (Nursing Council of New Zealand 2008c).

Nurses must be registered with the Nursing Council of New Zealand and hold a current **practising certificate** (renewed annually). Under the Trans Tasman Mutual Recognition (TTMR) Act, there is a reciprocal registration agreement with all states and territories of Australia (Nursing Council of New Zealand 2008d).

Since 2004, the Midwifery Council of New Zealand has been the statutory midwifery regulatory authority for midwives in New Zealand (Nursing Council of New Zealand 2008b).

QUESTION FOR REFLECTION

How is nursing regulated in your country and how does this compare to the regulation of nursing in New Zealand?

Types of nurses in New Zealand

In New Zealand, there are two levels of general nurse. A **registered nurse (RN)** must have a **Bachelor of Nursing (BN)** or equivalent qualification. The second-level nurse is referred to as a **nurse assistant** (as of 2004) or an **enrolled nurse (EN)** if the course was commenced or the nurse graduated between 2000 and 18 September 2004 (New Zealand Nurses Organisation 2007b) and must have a certificate acceptable for registration with the Nursing Council of New Zealand.

The New Zealand Nursing Council has five categories for registration: nurse practitioner; **nurse practitioner with prescribing rights**; registered nurse; enrolled nurse (not available for new registrants after 2004); and nurse assistant (since 2004) (Australian Nursing and Midwifery Council 2007k, Nursing Council of New Zealand 2008e). (See Table 4.4.)

In New Zealand, unregistered carers are referred to as healthcare assistants or support care workers and are sometimes employed in the aged care or disability sectors and in home care situations. These workers are *not* nurses.

TABLE 4.2 Professional nursing organisations and resources in Australia

Organisation	Purpose/mission	Sample resources/publications	Website
Australian Nursing and Midwifery Council (ANMC)	Peak body to facilitate a national approach to the regulation of nursing Develops national competency standards for nurses Develops position statements to assist policy development Develops guidelines for practice The International Section of the Australian Nursing and Midwifery Council (ANMC) is an assessing authority for the Australian Department of Immigration and Citizenship (DIAC) and determines suitability and education needs of overseas RNs and RMs who intend to migrate to Australia under the 'General Skilled Migration' category	Code of Ethics: June 2002 (with ANF, RCNA) Code of Professional Conduct, January 2003 National Competency Standards for the Registered Nurse, 4th edn, January 2006 National Competency Standards for the Midwife, 1st edn, January 2006 National Competency Standards for the Nurse Practitioner, 1st edn, January 2006 National Competency Standards for the Enrolled Nurse, October 2002 Principles for the Assessment of National Competency Standards, October 2002	www.anmc.org.au
Australian Nursing Federation (ANF)	National union for nurses Focuses on industrial and professional representation of nurses Develops policies, guidelines and position statements for nurses	Australian Nursing Journal (ANJ) Australian Journal of Advanced Nursing (AJAN) Code of Ethics, June 2002 (with ANMC, RCNA)	www.anf.org.au
Royal College of Nursing Australia (RCNA)	Peak national professional body representing all nurses. Promotes excellence in nursing though: • education • professional development	Collegian Nursing Review Code of Ethics, June 2002 (with ANF, ANMC)	www.rcna.org.au

(Continued)

TABLE 4.2 Professional nursing organisations and resources in Australia—*cont'd*

Organisation	Purpose/mission	Sample resources/publications	Website
Royal College of Nursing Australia (RCNA)—cont'd	• information and networking • contribution to health policy Representation on government committees and health advisory bodies Australian member of International Council of Nurses (ICN)		
Congress of Aboriginal and Torres Strait Islander Nurses (CATSIN)	Formally represents Indigenous nurses Focus on increasing numbers of Indigenous people in nursing	See website	www.indiginet.com.au/catsin
Australian Peak Nursing and Midwifery Forum (APNMF)	The following are members of this forum: ANMC, RCNA, ANF, CDNM, CATSIN and ACM	See websites of member organisations	See websites for member organisations
Australian College of Midwives (ACM)	Peak professional body for midwives	See website	www.acmi.org.au
Coalition of National Nursing Organisations (CoNNO) See ANF	Part of the ANF Coalition of nursing speciality organisations Represents specialties (e.g. stomal therapists, cardiovascular nurses, maternal and child health nurses)	See website	www.conno.org.au
Council of Deans of Nursing & Midwifery Australia and New Zealand (CDNM)	Peak body representing the Deans and Heads of the Schools of Nursing in universities that offer nursing and midwifery. Aims to: • ensure quality standards of education • be the 'voice' of tertiary education • lead and represent academics • promote the public image of nursing and midwifery	See website	www.cdnm.edu.au
National Enrolled Nurses Association (NENA) See ANF	Part of the ANF Represents and promotes the role of enrolled nurses	See website	ww.anf.org.au/NENA

TABLE 4.2 Professional nursing organisations and resources in Australia—*cont'd*

Organisation	Purpose/mission	Sample resources/publications	Website
Australian Nursing Regulatory Authorities	Regulatory authorities have the following responsibilities: • registration of nurses (including annual renewal of registration) • regulation of nursing (according to legislation) • accreditation of courses/education providers • ensuring the competence of nurses • protection of the public	See websites of the individual regulatory authorities for: • position statements • guidelines • codes • policies • other publications	See Table 4.3

Source: ACT Nursing and Midwifery Board 2007, Australian College of Midwives 2007, Australian Nursing and Midwifery Council 2007a, Australian Nursing Federation 2007, Congress of Aboriginal and Torres Strait Islander Nurses (CATSIN) 2007, Council of Deans of Nursing & Midwifery Australia and New Zealand 2007, Nurses and Midwives Board of NSW 2007, Nurses Board of South Australia 2007, Nurses Board of Victoria 2007, Nurses Board of Western Australia 2007, Nursing and Midwifery Board of Northern Territory 2007, Nursing Board of Tasmania 2007, Queensland Nursing Council 2007, Royal College of Nursing Australia 2007.

TABLE 4.3 Australian nursing regulatory authorities

State/ territory	Regulatory authority	Street address	Postal address	Telephone	Facsimile	Email	Website
Australian Capital Territory (ACT)	ACT Nursing and Midwifery Board	Suite 1 Scala House 11 Torrens St Braddon ACT 2612		61 2 6207 0413	61 2 6205 1602	actnmb@act.gov.au	www.nursesboard.act.gov.au
New South Wales (NSW)	Nurses and Midwives Board of NSW	Level 6 (North Wing) 477 Pitt Street Sydney NSW 2000	PO Box K599 Haymarket NSW 1238	61 2 9219 0222	61 2 9281 2030	mail@nmb.nsw.gov.au nmb@doh.health.nsw.gov.au	www.nmb.nsw.gov.au
Northern Territory (NT)	Nursing and Midwifery Board of Northern Territory	2nd Floor Harbour View Plaza cnr McMinns & Bennett Sts Darwin NT 0812	GPO Box 4221 Darwin NT 0801	61 8 8999 4157	61 8 8999 4196	healthprofessions.ths@nt.gov.au	www.nt.gov.au www.nt.gov.au/health/ registration boards/
Queensland (QLD)	Queensland Nursing Council	Level 14 201 Charlotte St Brisbane QLD 4000	GPO Box 292 Brisbane QLD 4001	61 7 3223 5111	61 7 3223 5115	executive@qnc.qld.gov.au general@qnc.qld.gov.au	www.qnc.qld.gov.au
South Australia (SA)	Nurses Board of South Australia	200 East Terrace Adelaide SA 5000	PO Box 7176 Hutt Street Adelaide SA 5000	61 8 8223 9700	61 8 8223 9707	registrations@nursesboard.sa.gov.au	www.nursesboard.sa.gov.au
Tasmania (TAS)	Nursing Board of Tasmania	151 Davey St Hobart Tas 7000	PO Box 847 Sandy Bay TAS 7006	61 3 6224 3991	61 3 6224 3995	nbt@nursingboardtas.com.au	www.nursingboardtas.org.au
Victoria (VIC)	Nurses Board of Victoria	Level 2 595 Little Collins St Melbourne VIC 3000	GPO Box 4932 Melbourne VIC 3001	61 3 8635 1200	61 3 8635 1248	registration@nbv.org.au	www.nbv.org.au

TABLE 4.3 Australian nursing regulatory authorities—*cont'd*

State/ territory	Regulatory authority	Street address	Postal address	Telephone	Facsimile	Email	Website
Western Australia (WA)	Nurses and Midwives Board of Western Australia	165 Adelaide Terrace East Perth WA 6892	Locked Bag 6 East Perth WA 6892	61 8 9421 1100	61 8 9421 1022	info@nmbwa.org.au	www.nmbwa.org.au

QUESTION FOR REFLECTION

What types of nurses are there in your country and how do they compare to the types of nurses in New Zealand?

Nursing education in New Zealand

In New Zealand, all teaching institutions (e.g. universities, polytechnics) who offer pre-registration nursing courses must be **accredited** by the national nursing regulatory authority (i.e. the Nursing Council of New Zealand). In addition, the course (which must include a clinical practice component, known as **clinical placement**) must be accredited by the Nursing Council of New Zealand. Registration as a nurse is only considered by the nursing regulatory authority for applicants who have successfully completed accredited courses at accredited institutions and passed the State Final Examination administered by the Nursing Council of New Zealand (Nursing Council of New Zealand 2008a).

In general, students must complete an approved Bachelor of Nursing course at a higher education institute to apply for registration as a registered nurse. Certificate courses for nurse assistants must be approved by the New Zealand Nursing Council and lead to a certificate at level 4 on the New Zealand Qualifications Authority—National Qualifications Framework (e.g. Certificate for Nurse Assistants, Certificate in Nursing) (Nursing Council of New Zealand 2008e).

Pre-registration nursing education courses provide a combination of theoretical and practical education. Pre-registration nursing courses include subjects (sometimes called units) from the sciences (including anatomy, physiology, pathophysiology, pharmacology), the social sciences (including psychology and sociology), law and ethics, and more recently specific units about cultural safety and Indigenous issues and health. Core nursing subjects address the history, theory and practice of nursing, and the professional issues relevant to nurses. Many courses also offer some elective subjects, so students have the opportunity to study an area that is of interest to them.

Students are required to undertake a broad range of clinical placements in healthcare settings such as hospitals, nursing homes, community health centres and mental health facilities. Clinical placement occurs throughout the course and students cannot be registered until the entire course has been successfully completed (unlike in some countries where a 2-year theoretical course is studied at college, followed by a 12-month clinical placement in a hospital). (Clinical placement is addressed in detail in Chs 12 and 13.)

There are many options for postgraduate nursing study. Nurses can study at the graduate certificate, graduate diploma, masters, and doctoral or PhD level. There are a number of models for postgraduate nursing education in the clinical **nursing speciality areas**, including critical care, emergency, perioperative, neurosciences, plastics and vascular, anaesthetics and recovery, aged care, maternal and child health, mental health and midwifery. Courses are offered by universities, often in conjunction with a hospital that provides the clinical placement and clinical education. Some nurses also undertake non-nursing postgraduate studies in disciplines such as education and management.

Table 4.4 compares the education and practice of the types of nurses in New Zealand.

TABLE 4.4 Nurses in New Zealand: classification, education and practice

Title	Educational qualification	Educational institute	Scope of practice	Notes
Registered nurse (RN)	Bachelor of Nursing (or equivalent): 3 years	University or polytechnics (since 1980s) Hospital (prior to early 1990)	Diverse areas, including specialties with further postgraduate education	
Former titles (registration under the *Nurses Act* 1977):			Scope of practice under the new HPCA Act (effective from 18 September 2004)	All of these nurses are classified as registered nurses (but their scopes of practice are restricted as listed)
Registered comprehensive nurse			As per current RN	
Registered general and obstetric nurse			May practise only in general and obstetric nursing	
Registered psychiatric nurse			May practise only in mental health nursing	
Registered psychopaedic nurse			May practise only in settings that provide services for consumers with intellectual disabilities	
Registered general nurse			May practise only in general nursing	
Registered obstetric nurse			May practise only within a maternity setting under the direction of a midwife or a medical practitioner	

(Continued)

TABLE 4.4 Nurses in New Zealand: classification, education and practice—*cont'd*

Title	Educational qualification	Educational institute	Scope of practice	Notes
Nurse practitioner	Bachelor of Nursing Master's degree in specialty area of nursing (*and* demonstrated clinical expertise)	University or polytechnics	May practise only within a specific designated area of practice	
Nurse practitioner with prescribing rights	Bachelor of Nursing Master's degree in specialty area of nursing (*and* demonstrated clinical expertise)	University or polytechnics	May practise and prescribe only within a specific designated area of practice	
Nurse assistant (since 18 September 2004) Formerly: Enrolled nurse (educated before 2000) Enrolled nurse (if course was commenced or graduated between 2000 and 18 September 2004)	Certificate (approved by NZ Nursing Council) at level 4 on the New Zealand Qualifications Authority—National Qualifications Framework (e.g. Certificate for Nurse Assistants, Certificate in Nursing)	Various	Restricted practice Second-level nurse Various areas (usually excluding acute specialties)	As of 4 July 2007, these nurses have been titled 'enrolled nurses', not 'nurse assistants', after the NZNO won an appeal to the Parliament's Regulations Review Committee

Source: New Zealand Nurses Organisation 2007b, Nursing Council of New Zealand 2008e.

?

QUESTION FOR REFLECTION

How does nursing education in your country compare with nursing education in New Zealand?

Professional nursing organisations and resources in New Zealand

There are various nursing organisations and resources in New Zealand (see Table 4.5). It is important to be familiar with the nursing regulatory authority and with the professional bodies that represent nursing.

CHAPTER HIGHLIGHTS

- Nurses in Australia and New Zealand are generally well respected and trusted health professionals.
- Nurses in Australia and New Zealand work in a diverse range of settings in urban, rural and remotes areas.
- Nurses in Australia and New Zealand work in a diverse range of roles, including as clinicians, educators, academics, researchers, managers, consultants and leaders.
- In both Australia and New Zealand, the term nurse practitioner refers to a nurse who has very advanced knowledge, skills and education in a speciality area of practice, and may have prescribing rights. Nurse practitioners must be registered as such. The term does not simply refer to a nurse in clinical practice.
- In Australia and New Zealand, nurse workloads are determined by the nurse–patient ratio method or predicted using a patient dependency system.
- In both Australia and New Zealand, nursing regulatory authorities govern the practice of nursing, and nurses are required by law to be registered with the relevant nursing regulatory authority.
- In both Australia and New Zealand, the nursing regulatory authorities must accredit teaching institutions and nursing courses.
- The two levels of general nurse in Australia are registered nurse (or registered nurse Div 1 in Victoria) and enrolled nurse (or registered nurse Div 2 in Victoria).
- In Australia, registered nurses (or registered nurses Div 1 in Victoria) must have a Bachelor of Nursing degree or equivalent from an accredited tertiary institution, and enrolled nurses (or registered nurses Div 2 in Victoria) must have a certificate or diploma from an accredited provider, often a TAFE institute. After successful course completion, nurses are eligible to apply for registration.
- The two levels of general nurse in New Zealand are registered nurse and nurse assistant (or enrolled nurse if the course was commenced or the nurse graduated between 2000 and 18 September 2004).
- In New Zealand, registered nurses must have a Bachelor of Nursing degree or equivalent from an accredited tertiary institution, and nurse assistants must have a relevant certificate (at level 4 on the New Zealand Qualifications Authority—National Qualifications Framework) from an accredited provider. After successful course completion, and passing the State Final Examination administered by the Nursing Council of New Zealand, nurses are eligible to apply for registration.
- Various statutory bodies and professional nursing organisations exist in both Australia and New Zealand, and provide valuable resources for nurses.

TABLE 4.5 Professional nursing organisations and resources in New Zealand

Organisation	Purpose/mission	Sample resources/ publications	Website
College of Nurses Aotearoa New Zealand (CNA–NZ)	Peak professional body representing all nurses Promotes excellence in nursing through: • promoting professional development (in clinical practice, nursing management, nursing education and research) • monitoring and advising on education • providing information • promoting and publishing nursing/health research • contribution to health policy Provides a 'voice' for nurses	Te Puawai Nursing Praxis	www.nurse.org.nz
Council of Deans of Nursing & Midwifery Australia and New Zealand (CDNM)	Peak body representing the Deans and Heads of the Schools of Nursing in universities that offer nursing and midwifery. Aims to: • ensure quality standards of education • be the 'voice' of tertiary education • lead and represent academics • promote the public image of nursing and midwifery	See website	www.cdnm.edu.au
New Zealand College of Midwives	Peak professional body for midwives	See website	www.midwife.org.nz
New Zealand Nurses Organisation (NZNO)	Professional nursing organisation National union for nurses, midwives and hospital aides Focuses on industrial and professional representation of nurses Contributes to health policy, nursing policy, nursing education and the organisation of health services	Kai Tiaki Nursing New Zealand	www.nzno.org.nz

TABLE 4.5 Professional nursing organisations and resources in New Zealand—*cont'd*

Organisation	Purpose/mission	Sample resources/ publications	Website
New Zealand Nurses Organisation (NZNO)—cont'd	Develops pamphlets, policies, position statements and guidelines, papers and handbooks Works according to the Treaty of Waitangi or Te Tiriti o Waitangi New Zealand member of International Council of Nurses (ICN)		
NZNO National Enrolled Nurse Section See NZNO	Part of the NZNO Represents and promotes the role of enrolled nurses	See website	www.nzno.org.nz/Site/Sections/Sections/Enrolled_Nurses
Nursing Council of New Zealand or Te Kaunihera o Aotearoa	Regulatory authority for New Zealand nurses Responsibilities: • registration of nurses (including annual renewal of registration) • regulation of nursing (according to legislation) • accreditation of courses/education providers • ensuring the competence of nurses • protection of the public	Code of Conduct for Nurses, March 2008 Competencies for Registered Nurses, December 2007 Competencies for Nurse Assistants and Enrolled Nurses, December 2007 Nurse Practitioner Competencies (undated, review pending) Guidelines for Cultural Safety, the Treaty of Waitangi, and Māori Health in Nursing Education and Practice, March 2005 Annual reports (see website)	www.nursingcouncil.org.nz
Te Kaunihera O Nga Neehi Māori O Aotearoa or National Council of Māori Nurses	Represents Māori with respect to health (and is mandated to do so) Focuses on workforce development Works with other Māori and nursing bodies	See website	www.maorihealth.co.nz www.maorihealth.co.nz/index.php
—	—	New Zealand Nursing Review	www.nursingreview.co.nz

Source: College of Nurses Aotearoa New Zealand 2007, Council of Deans of Nursing & Midwifery Australia and New Zealand 2007, National Council of Māori Nurses 2007, New Zealand College of Midwives 2007, New Zealand Nurses Organisation 2007a, Nursing Council of New Zealand 2008c.

Self-test questions

Plain numbered questions are for all readers; 'a' questions are for readers in Australia; 'b' questions are for readers in New Zealand.

1a. Go to the following website: www.anmc.org.au/wpsear/country_profiles.php. Use the link to your country and the link to the state or territory in Australia where you are working or studying. List the similarities and differences between nursing in your country and nursing in the state or territory in Australia where you are studying or working.

1b. Go to the following website: www.anmc.org.au/wpsear/country_profiles.php. Use the link to your country and the link to New Zealand. List the similarities and differences between nursing in your country and nursing in New Zealand.

2. What is the name of the law that governs the practice of nurses where you are working or studying?

3. Review the website of the nursing regulatory authority where you are working or studying, and discuss its role.

4a. Briefly describe the educational qualifications, course education providers and scopes of practice for the following: registered nurse/registered nurse (Div 1); enrolled nurse/registered nurse (Div 2); nurse practitioner; and midwife.

4b. Briefly describe the educational qualifications, course education providers and scopes of practice for the following: registered nurse; enrolled nurse; nurse assistant; nurse practitioner; and nurse practitioner with prescribing rights.

5. Describe the role of the nursing regulatory authority where you are working or studying, with respect to nursing education.

6a. Read and summarise a recent journal article about nurse practitioners in Australia using the 'Article summary sheet' (R1) on the CD Part 3—Reader resources.

6b. Read and summarise a recent journal article about nurse practitioners in New Zealand using the 'Article summary sheet' (R1) on the CD Part 3—Reader resources.

7a. Read and summarise a recent journal article about remote area nursing in Australia using the 'Article summary sheet' (R1) on the CD Part 3—Reader resources.

7b. Read and summarise a recent journal article about remote area nursing in New Zealand using the 'Article summary sheet' (R1) on the CD Part 3—Reader resources.

8. Review the key terms and any other new vocabulary, terms and abbreviations from this chapter, and then update your 'Language list' (R2) on the CD Part 3—Reader resources.

9. Answer the 'Learning objectives' at the start of this chapter as if they were examination questions.

References

ACT Nursing and Midwifery Board 2007 ACT Nursing and Midwifery Board. Online. Available www.actnmb.act.gov.au/index.html 1 July 2007

Australian College of Midwives 2007 Welcome. Online. Available www.acmi.org.au 12 July 2007

Australian Nursing and Midwifery Council 2006 National Competency standards for the Nurse Practitioner. Online. Available www.anmc.org.au/docs/Competency_Standards_for_the_Nurse_Practitioner.pdf 2 Aug 2007

Australian Nursing and Midwifery Council 2007a About ANMC. Online. Available www.anmc.org.au/about/index.php 2 Aug 2007

Australian Nursing and Midwifery Council 2007b Australia: Australian Capital Territory. Online. Available www.anmc.org.au/wpsear/ACT.php 2 Aug 2007
Australian Nursing and Midwifery Council 2007c Australia: New South Wales. Online. Available www.anmc.org.au/wpsear/NSW.php 2 Aug 2007
Australian Nursing and Midwifery Council 2007d Australia: Northern Territory. Online. Available www.anmc.org.au/wpsear/NT.php 2 Aug 2007
Australian Nursing and Midwifery Council 2007e Australia: Queensland. Online. Available www.anmc.org.au/wpsear/QLD.php 2 Aug 2007
Australian Nursing and Midwifery Council 2007f Australia: South Australia. Online. Available www.anmc.org.au/wpsear/SA.php 2 Aug 2007
Australian Nursing and Midwifery Council 2007g Australia: Tasmania. Online. Available www.anmc.org.au/wpsear/TAS.php 2 Aug 2007
Australian Nursing and Midwifery Council 2007h Australia: Victoria. Online. Available www.anmc.org.au/wpsear/VIC.php 2 Aug 2007
Australian Nursing and Midwifery Council 2007i Australia: Western Australia. Online. Available www.anmc.org.au/wpsear/WA.php 2 Aug 2007
Australian Nursing and Midwifery Council 2007j Country profiles for the nursing and midwifery regulatory authorities of the Western Pacific and South East Asian regions. Online. Available www.anmc.org.au/wpsear/country_profiles.php 2 Aug 2007
Australian Nursing and Midwifery Council 2007k New Zealand. Online. Available www.anmc.org.au/wpsear/NZ.php 2 Aug 2007
Australian Nursing and Midwifery Council 2007l Welcome to Australian Nursing and Midwifery Council Incorporated (ANMC). Online. Available www.anmc.org.au/index.php 2 Aug 2007
Australian Nursing Federation 2007 About ANF. Online. Available www.anf.org.au 12 July 2007
College of Nurses Aotearoa New Zealand 2007 About us. Online. Available www.nurse.org.nz/about.htm 8 July 2007
Congress of Aboriginal and Torres Strait Islander Nurses (CATSIN) 2007 Preamble. Online. Available www.indiginet.com.au/catsin/preamble.html 12 July 2007
Council of Australian Governments 2008a Council of Australian Governments' Communique, 26 March 2008. Online. Available www.coag.gov.au/meetings/ 130407/ 12 May 2008
Council of Australian Governments 2008b Intergovernmental agreement for a national registration and accreditation scheme for the health professions. Online. Available www.coag.gov.au/meetings/260308/docs/iga_health_workforce.rtf / 12 May 2008
Council of Deans of Nursing & Midwifery Australia and New Zealand 2007 Introduction. Online. Available www.cdnm.edu.au/intro.html 19 July 2007
National Council of Māori Nurses 2007 Welcome to the web site of Te Kauniera O Nga Neehi Maori O Aotearoa. Online. Available www.maorihealth.co.nz/ 31 July 2007
New Zealand College of Midwives 2007 New Zealand College of Midwives. Online. Available www.midwife.org.nz 19 July 2007
New Zealand Ministry of Health 2006 Health Practitioners Competence Assurance Act 2003. Online. Available www.moh.govt.nz/hpca 12 May 2007
New Zealand Nurses Organisation 2007a About NZNO. Online. Available www.nzno.org.nz/Site/About/about.aspx 17 July 2007
New Zealand Nurses Organisation 2007b Good news for many enrolled nurses. Online. Available www.nzno.org.nz/Site/News/Latest/EN.aspx 6 July 2007
Nurses and Midwives Board of NSW 2007 Welcome. Online. Available www.nmb.nsw.gov.au 2 July 2007
Nurses Board of South Australia 2007 Welcome. Online. Available www.nursesboard.sa.gov.au/index.html 2 July 2007

Nurses Board of Victoria 2007 About the Nurses Board of Victoria. Online. Available www.nbv.org.au/about-us.aspx 2 July 2007
Nurses Board of Western Australia 2007 Welcome to the Board. Online. Available www.nbwa.org.au/1/1096/50/welcome_to_the_.pm 2 July 2007
Nursing and Midwifery Board of Northern Territory 2007 Health professions licensing authority: Nursing and midwifery board. Online. Available www.nt.gov.au/health/org_supp/prof_boards/nurse_midwifery/board.shtml 2 July 2007
Nursing Board of Tasmania 2007 About the Nursing Board of Tasmania. Online. Available www.nursingboardtas.org.au/nbtonline.nsf/$LookupDocName/about_the_nurses_board_of_tasmania 2 July 2007
Nursing Council of New Zealand 2008a Education. Online. Available www.nursingcouncil.org.nz/educa.html 13 May 2008
Nursing Council of New Zealand 2008b Midwifery. Online. Available www.nursingcouncil.org.nz/midwifery.html 13 May 2008
Nursing Council of New Zealand 2008c Nursing Council of New Zealand. Online. Available www.nursingcouncil.org.nz/ 13 May 2008
Nursing Council of New Zealand 2008d Registration in New Zealand for nurses from overseas. Online. Available www.nursingcouncil.org.nz/reg.html 13 May 2008
Nursing Council of New Zealand 2008e Scopes of practice. Online. Available www.nursingcouncil.org.nz/scopes.html#nas 13 May 2008
O'Connor T 2006 Do nurse/patient ratios work? Kai Tiaki Nursing New Zealand 12(3):12–14
Plummer V 2005 Accounting for nurse staffing resources. Paper presented at RCNA Annual Conference, July 2005, Adelaide, Australia. Online. Available www.rcna.org.au/UserFiles/virginia_plummer_4b_pages_1-22.pdf 21 Feb 2008
Queensland Nursing Council 2007 About the QNC. Online. Available www.qnc.qld.gov.au/home/content.aspx?content=About_the_QNC/About_the_QNC 2 July 2007
Royal College of Nursing Australia 2007 About RCNA. Online. Available www.rcna.org.au/site/aboutrcna.php 20 July 2007

CHAPTER 5

Nursing standards and competencies

'Nursing is different from in my country. Nurses are very responsible for everything here. Nurses must have great knowledge, and also do many skills. Always we must be competent.'

Yik Fai, China

CHAPTER OUTLINE

LEARNING OBJECTIVES

1. Discuss the regulation of nursing in Australia or New Zealand.
2. Discuss the Australian or New Zealand regulatory frameworks for nursing.
3. Discuss the relevant codes of ethics and/or conduct for nurses in Australia or New Zealand.
4. Describe the history and purpose of the relevant competency standards in Australia or New Zealand.
5. Discuss the meaning of the terms 'competence' and 'competent'.
6. Outline the structure of the relevant competency standards in Australia or New Zealand.

7. Discuss in detail the core competency standards for all nurses in Australia or New Zealand.
8. Identify the key standards and competencies-related resources for nurses in Australia or New Zealand.

Key terms (are in bold in the text)

audit
Australian Nursing and Midwifery Council (ANMC)
Code of Conduct for Nurses (NZ)
Code of Ethics for Nurses in Australia
Code of Professional Conduct for Nurses in Australia
competence
competencies for nurses (formerly competencies for the scopes of practice) (NZ)
competency/competencies
competency elements (Aus)
competency units (Aus)
competent
Continuing Competence Framework (NZ)
cues (Aus)
cultural competence
cultural safety (NZ)
domains
Health Practitioners Competence Assurance Act (HPCAA) (NZ)
indicators (NZ)
National Competency Standards (Aus)
National Continuing Competence Framework (Draft 3) (Aus)
National Continuing Competence Project (Aus)
Nursing Council of New Zealand
nursing regulatory authorities
portfolio
practice hours
professional development
professional misconduct
recertification (audit) programme (NZ)
registration
standards
Treaty of Waitangi (NZ)
unprofessional conduct

In Australia and New Zealand, nursing standards and competencies are considered to be of critical importance in ensuring that nurses are competent professionals. While each country has its own published standards and competencies, there are many similarities in the expectations of nurses in both countries. To study and practise nursing in Australia or New Zealand, you will need to be familiar with the standards and competencies of the profession. It is essential for all nurses to meet the legislative requirements for registration and practice. This includes meeting the profession's ethical, professional conduct and competency standards. It is also important for nurses to be able to provide evidence of their continuing competence.

Nursing standards and competencies in Australia

Nursing regulation, standards and competencies

While there are currently separate state and territory laws that govern the practice of nursing (with a proposed national system due to commence in 2010, which will see a single national nursing regulatory authority responsible for the **registration** and regulation of nursing) (Council of Australian Governments 2008a, 2008b), all legislation requires nurses to be safe and **competent**, and to meet the profession's **standards** and **competencies**.

The **nursing regulatory authorities** in each state and territory are the statutory bodies that govern nursing in Australia. All of the nursing regulatory authorities have adopted the **Code of Ethics for Nurses in Australia**, the **Code of Professional Conduct for Nurses in Australia** and the **National Competency Standards** published by the **Australian Nursing and Midwifery Council (ANMC)**. These documents—along with the position statements and guidelines published by the ANMC and the individual nursing regulatory authorities—are part of the regulatory framework for nursing in Australia (Australian Nursing and Midwifery Council 2006 p 1, 2002 p 2). It is anticipated that the **National Continuing Competence Framework** (Australian Nursing and Midwifery Council 2008a, Australian Nursing and Midwifery Council 2008b), which is currently being developed, will also form part of this regulatory framework by the end of 2008.

The Code of Ethics 'focuses on the ethics and ideals of the profession [and] the Code of Professional Conduct identifies the minimum requirements for practice in the profession' (Australian Nursing and Midwifery Council 2002a p 2). The National Competency Standards reflect the competencies required of nurses who are registered or seeking registration in Australia (Australian Nursing and Midwifery Council 2006 p 1).

Code of Ethics

The Code of Ethics for Nurses in Australia 'outlines the profession's intention to accept the rights of individuals and uphold these rights in practice' (Australian Nursing and Midwifery Council 2002a p 1). See Table 5.1.

TABLE 5.1 The Code of Ethics for Nurses in Australia

The purpose of the Code of Ethics is to: • identify the fundamental moral commitments of the profession • provide nurses with a basis for professional and self-reflection on ethical conduct • act as a guide to ethical practice, and • indicate to the community the moral values which nurses can be expected to hold.
The Code of Ethics contains six value statements: 1. Nurses respect individuals' needs, values, culture and vulnerability in the provision of nursing care. 2. Nurses accept the rights of individuals to make informed choices in relation to their healthcare. 3. Nurses promote and uphold the provision of quality nursing care for all people. 4. Nurses hold in confidence any information obtained in a professional capacity, use professional judgment where there is a need to share information for the therapeutic benefit and safety of a person and ensure that privacy is safeguarded. 5. Nurses fulfil the accountability and responsibility inherent in their roles. 6. Nurses value environmental ethics and a social, economic and ecologically sustainable environment that promotes health and wellbeing.

Source: Australian Nursing and Midwifery Council 2002a pp 1, 3–5.

Code of Professional Conduct

The Code of Professional Conduct for Nurses in Australia is 'a set of expected national standards of nursing conduct [whereby] a breach may constitute **professional misconduct** or **unprofessional conduct**' (Australian Nursing and Midwifery Council 2003 p 1) and lead to deregistration. See Table 5.2.

TABLE 5.2 The Code of Professional Conduct for Nurses in Australia

The purpose of the Code of Professional Conduct is to: • set an expected national standard of conduct for the nursing profession • inform the community of the standards for professional conduct of nurses in Australia, and • provide consumer, regulatory, employing and professional bodies with a basis for decisions regarding standards of professional conduct.
The Code of Professional Conduct contains nine statements and stipulates that: 1. A nurse must practise in a safe and competent manner. 2. A nurse must practise in accordance with the agreed standards of the profession. 3. A nurse must not bring discredit upon the reputation of the nursing profession. 4. A nurse must practise in accordance with laws relevant to the nurse's area of practice. 5. A nurse must respect the dignity, culture, values and beliefs of an individual and any significant other person. 6. A nurse must support the health, wellbeing and informed decision making of an individual. 7. A nurse must promote and preserve the trust that is inherent in the privileged relationship between a nurse and an individual and respect both the person and property of the individual. 8. A nurse must treat personal information obtained in a professional capacity as confidential. 9. A nurse must refrain from engaging in exploitation, misinformation or misrepresentation in regard to healthcare products and nursing services.

Source: Australian Nursing and Midwifery Council 2003 pp 1, 2–4.

QUESTION FOR REFLECTION

How do the Code of Ethics for Nurses in Australia and the Code of Professional Conduct for Nurses in Australia compare to the standards for ethics and conduct for nurses in your country?

National Competency Standards

History

In 1990, the Australian Nurse Registering Authorities Conference (ANRAC) initially developed competencies for registered nurses in Australia. The successor organisation was the Australian Nursing Council Incorporated (ANCI), which, along with all of the Australian nursing regulatory authorities, adopted these standards. In 2004, ANCI became the Australian Nursing and Midwifery Council (ANMC). Since their inception, the competency standards have been reviewed and updated a number of times, and competency standards for enrolled nurses, midwives and nurse practitioners have been developed.

Currently, the National Competency Standards available are:

- the National Competency Standards for the Registered Nurse, 4th edn, January 2006
- the National Competency Standards for the Midwife, 1st edn, January 2006
- the National Competency Standards for the Nurse Practitioner, 1st edn, January 2006, and
- the National Competency Standards for the Enrolled Nurse, 2002 (review pending).

Purpose and applications

The National Competency Standards are essentially a benchmark providing a standard against which a nurse's performance is measured. There are guidelines to assist managers and educators in the use of the standards to assess nurses' competence (Australian Nursing and Midwifery Council 2002c). The standards can be used in the following ways:

- to determine whether an applicant is competent and fit for initial registration or re-registration (this applies to recent graduates, overseas nurses and former nurses who want to re-enter the profession)
- to determine whether an applicant is competent and fit for renewal of registration—in states and territories where the legislation allows competence assessment for continuing registration (e.g. in some states and territories, nurses must sign an annual declaration attesting to their competence as per the National Competency Standards, before a renewal of registration certificate is issued)
- to assess clinical performance in the academic setting (e.g. used as an assessment tool during clinical placement)
- to assess performance in the workplace (e.g. used as a tool for annual workplace performance reviews), and
- to assess performance in the workplace where the nurse's fitness to practise is being assessed (e.g. a nurse who is being assessed due to poor performance or professional conduct matters).

In addition, the standards communicate to the general public—and other health professionals—the standards and competencies expected of nurses (Australian Nursing and Midwifery Council 2006 p 1).

Registration and competence

In August 2007, the **National Continuing Competence Project** commenced in Australia, and a National Continuing Competence Framework was drafted (Australian Nursing and Midwifery Council 2008a, Australian Nursing and Midwifery Council 2008b). It is anticipated that the project will be completed in 2008. As part of the proposed National Continuing Competence Framework, it is expected that all nurses and midwives who are applying to register, re-register or renew their registration will be competent—and able to provide evidence of their competence (Australian Nursing and Midwifery Council 2008a).

Nurses seeking renewal of registration will be expected to maintain a **portfolio** detailing their continuing competence over the preceding 3 years. It is anticipated that it will be mandatory for nurses and midwives to meet continuing competency requirements, before being eligible for applying to the nursing regulatory authority for renewal of registration (Australian Nursing and Midwifery Council 2008b p 2). The specific continuing competence requirements proposed are:

- assessment (annual self-assessment based on ANMC competency standards, professional review and annual self-declaration of competence)
- **practice hours** (minimum 420 over 3 years)
- continuing **professional development** (CPD) (30 hours per year), and
- portfolio (to contain evidence of continuing competency activities) (Australian Nursing and Midwifery Council 2008b p 5).

It is proposed that nursing regulatory authorities will conduct annual audits of 5% of nurses before their registration is renewed, and, if requested, nurses must be able to produce evidence of their continuing competence from their portfolios (Australian Nursing and Midwifery Council 2008b p 13). The **National Continuing Competence Framework (Draft 2)** contains information about portfolio development for nurses (Australian Nursing and Midwifery Council 2008b p 7).

Sample portfolio templates are available from the Nurses and Midwives Board of Western Australia (2007), and a sample record of professional development activities is available from the Australian Nursing Federation (2008). It is also recommended that you read a text that addresses portfolio development, listed in the 'Recommended reading' (Andre & Heartfield 2006). Always ensure that your portfolio contains the relevant evidence to meet the continuing competency requirements for renewal of your registration.

Defining competence

It is essential for you to fully understand the competency standards, as you will be assessed according to these standards. To do so, you will need to understand the meaning of the terms competence and competent. **Competence** is 'the combination of skills, knowledge, attitudes, values and abilities that underpin effective and/or superior performance in a profession/occupational area' (Australian Nursing and Midwifery Council 2006 p 8). **Competent** means 'the person has competence across all the domains of competencies applicable to the nurse, at a standard that is judged to be appropriate for the level of nurse being assessed' (Australian Nursing and Midwifery Council 2006 p 8).

It is very important to note that competence is not simply 'doing' a skill, or 'getting the work done', and it includes your skills, knowledge, attitudes, values and abilities. To be considered competent, you will need to demonstrate your competence in *all* the domains or aspects of nursing practice. (The assessment of competence during clinical placement is addressed in detail in Ch 13.)

Cultural competence

In Australian nursing practice, **cultural competence** is not a discrete competency standard, but is implicit in the Code of Ethics for Nurses in Australia (Australian Nursing and Midwifery Council 2002a), the Code of Professional Conduct for Nurses in Australia (Australian Nursing and Midwifery Council 2003) and the National Competency Standards for Nurses (Australian Nursing and Midwifery Council 2002b, 2006). It is important for nurses in Australia to understand the issues associated with culture and ethnicity and their impact on health, and it is highly recommended that you read about these concepts in the source listed in the 'Recommended reading' (Dowd et al 2009).

An understanding of the New Zealand perspective on cultural safety, cultural competence and nursing is helpful for nurses in Australia. **Cultural safety** is a very important concept in New Zealand nursing practice, and is a core competency for all nurses (Nursing Council of New Zealand 2007a p 7, 2007b p 9). Cultural safety is defined as:

> . . . the effective nursing practice of a person from another culture, and is determined by that person or family [and requires that] the nurse delivering the nursing service will have

> undertaken a process of reflection on his or her own cultural identity and will recognise [its] impact . . . on professional practice (Nursing Council of New Zealand 2005 p 7).

Chapter 6 specifically addresses these concepts in New Zealand nursing practice.

Structure of the National Competency Standards

The ANMC National Competency Standards for both registered and enrolled nurses are structured according to four **domains** that are major aspects, areas or parameters of nursing practice. Within each domain are a number of **competency units** that are separate functional areas (and are effectively individual competencies). Each competency unit has a number of **competency elements** that are parts of the competency unit. **Cues** or examples are provided for each competency element to represent competent performance. Tables 5.3 and 5.4 outline the key aspects of each domain for the registered nurse and the enrolled nurse (Table 5.4 also applies to registered nurses Div 2 in Victoria).

> ? **QUESTION FOR REFLECTION**
> How do the National Competency Standards compare to the competency standards for nurses in your country?

Required resources

You will need to obtain copies of the documents listed in Table 5.5.

Nursing standards and competencies in New Zealand

Nursing regulation, standards and competencies

The **Health Practitioners Competence Assurance Act (HPCAA) 2003** requires nurses to be safe and competent, and to meet the profession's standards and competencies (New Zealand Ministry of Health 2006, Nursing Council of New Zealand 2008b).

The **Nursing Council of New Zealand** or Te Kaunihera Tapuhi o Aotearoa is the statutory nursing authority that governs the practice of nurses in New Zealand. The HPCAA 'requires the Council to ensure the continuing **competence** of practitioners to protect public safety' (Nursing Council of New Zealand 2008b).

The Nursing Council of New Zealand has developed a **Continuing Competence Framework** to ensure nurses are suitable for initial registration and renewal of registration. The framework requires all nurses to provide evidence of their competence, professional development activities and practice hours.

The Nursing Council of New Zealand has a **Code of Conduct for Nurses** and has developed competencies for the registered nurse, nurse assistant and enrolled nurse, along with nurse practitioner **competencies**, as part of the regulatory framework for nursing in New Zealand.

The Code of Conduct identifies 'the minimum **standards** expected of nurses' (Nursing Council of New Zealand 2008a p 2). The **competencies for nurses** reflect the competencies required of all nurses who are registered or seeking registration in New Zealand (Nursing Council of New Zealand 2008b).

TABLE 5.3 National Competency Standards for the Registered Nurse in Australia: overview of the domains

Domain	Key aspects (reflected by the competency units and elements)
Professional practice	Professional, legal, ethical responsibilities Knowledge base (for safe practice) Accountability and recognition of own scope of practice Abiding by legislation Protection of human rights (includes concepts such as: respect, dignity, cultural sensitivity, advocacy, privacy, confidentiality)
Critical thinking and analysis	Self-assessment Professional development Valuing evidence and research Reflective practice (including the awareness of the impact of 'self' on others)
Provision and coordination of care	Coordination, organisation, provision of care Time management Prioritisation Use of the nursing process: assessment, planning, implementation and evaluation of nursing care
Collaborative and therapeutic practice	Therapeutic relationship management: • communication • information/education • advocacy • maintaining safety and security (including cultural safety) Interdisciplinary team member skills: • supervision and delegation • coordination and management of care

Source: Australian Nursing and Midwifery Council 2006.

Code of Conduct

The Code of Conduct for Nurses is a set of principles with criteria outlining the 'minimum standards expected of nurses' (Nursing Council of New Zealand 2008a p 2), whereby a breach may constitute **professional misconduct** and lead to penalties, including deregistration. See Table 5.6.

?

QUESTION FOR REFLECTION

How does the Code of Conduct compare to the standards of conduct for nurses in your country?

Competencies for nurses

History

To meet its obligations under the Health Practitioners Competence Assurance Act, the Nursing Council of New Zealand introduced **competencies for the scopes of practice** for nurses in 2005, which were updated in 2007, and are now referred to as competencies

TABLE 5.4 National Competency Standards for the Enrolled Nurse in Australia: overview of the domains

Domain	Key aspects (reflected by the competency units and elements)
Professional and ethical practice	Professional, legal, ethical responsibilities Knowledge base (for safe practice) Accountability and recognition of own scope of practice Abiding by legislation Protection of human rights (includes concepts such as: respect, dignity, cultural sensitivity, advocacy, privacy, confidentiality)
Critical thinking and analysis	Self-assessment Professional development Self-care Reflective practice (including the awareness of the impact of 'self' on others)
Management of care	Time management Data gathering and reporting Under the supervision of the registered nurse (or RN Div 1 in Victoria), use of the nursing process: assessment, planning, implementation and evaluation of nursing care
Enabling	Communication Information/education Promoting safety and security

Source: Australian Nursing and Midwifery Council 2002b.

TABLE 5.5 Resources for overseas nurses and international nursing students in Australia

Student/nurse	Document	Source
All nursing students and nurses	Code of Ethics for Nurses in Australia, 2002	www.anmc.org.au/docs/ANMC_Code_of_Ethics.pdf
	Code of Professional Conduct for Nurses in Australia, 2003	www.anmc.org.au/docs/ANMC_Professional_Conduct.pdf
Bachelor of Nursing students Registered nurse/registered nurses (Div 1)	National Competency Standards for the Registered Nurse, 4th edn, January 2006	www.anmc.org.au/docs/Competency_standards_RN.pdf
	National Competency Standards for the Enrolled Nurse, October 2002 (review pending)	www.anmc.org.au/docs/Publications/Competency%20standards%20EN.pdf
Registered nurses/registered nurses (Div 1): Nurse educators, managers, researchers, leaders	National Competency Standards for the Registered Nurse, 4th edn, January 2006	www.anmc.org.au/docs/Competency_standards_RN.pdf
	Principles for the Assessment of National Competency Standards, October 2002	www.anmc.org.au/docs/Principles%20for%20the%20Assessment.pdf
Certificate IV in Health/Certificate IV in Nursing/Diploma in Nursing students Enrolled nurses/registered nurses (Div 2)	National Competency Standards for the Enrolled Nurse, October 2002 (review pending)	www.anmc.org.au/docs/Publications/Competency%20standards%20EN.pdf

TABLE 5.6 The Code of Conduct for Nurses in New Zealand

The purpose of the Code of Conduct for Nurses is to provide a guide: • for the public to assess minimum standards expected of nurses, and • for nurses to monitor their own performance and that of their colleagues.
The Code of Conduct for Nurses contains four principles and stipulates that the nurse: 1. complies with legislated requirements 2. acts ethically and maintains standards of practice 3. respects the rights of patients/clients, and 4. justifies public trust and confidence.

Source: Nursing Council of New Zealand 2008a pp 2–6.

for nurses. These competencies are part of the Council's **Continuing Competence Framework**. The competencies available are: the Competencies for Registered Nurses, December 2007; the Competencies for Nurse Assistants and Enrolled Nurses, December 2007; and the Nurse Practitioner Competencies (undated; review pending).

Purpose and applications

The competencies for nurses are essentially a benchmark providing a standard against which a nurse's performance is measured. They can be used:

- to determine whether an applicant is competent and fit for initial registration or re-registration (this applies to recent graduates, overseas nurses and former nurses who want to re-enter the profession)
- to determine whether an applicant is competent and fit for renewal of registration—continuing competence is a legislated requirement in New Zealand (and nurses are expected to maintain evidence of their continuing competence which could be audited) (Nursing Council of New Zealand 2006a, 2006b, 2008d)
- to assess clinical performance in the academic setting (e.g. used as an assessment tool during clinical placement)
- to assess performance in the workplace (e.g. used as a tool for annual workplace performance review), and
- to assess performance in the workplace where the nurse's fitness to practise is being assessed (e.g. a nurse who is being assessed due to poor performance or professional conduct matters).

In addition, national competency standards communicate to the general public—and other health professionals—the standards and competencies expected of nurses (Australian Nursing and Midwifery Council 2006 p 1).

Registration and competence

As part of the Nursing Council of New Zealand's **Continuing Competence Framework**, it is expected that all nurses who are applying to register, re-register or renew their registration will be competent—and able to provide evidence of their competence (Nursing Council of New Zealand 2008b).

Nurses seeking renewal of their annual practising certificates are expected to maintain a **portfolio** detailing their continuing competence over the preceding 3 years. The specific continuing competence requirements are:

- **practice hours** (minimum 450 hours over the last 3 years)
- **professional development** activities (minimum 60 hours over the last 3 years), and
- meeting all of the **competencies** for the relevant scope of practice and completing the Nursing Council of New Zealand's competence assessment form (two of these three methods must be used: self-assessment, peer review, assessment by senior nurse) (Nursing Council of New Zealand 2008d).

As part of its **recertification (audit) programme**, each year the Nursing Council of New Zealand audits 5% of nurses before their annual practising certificates are issued, and, if requested, nurses must be able to produce evidence of their continuing competence from their portfolios (Nursing Council of New Zealand 2008d). Information about portfolio development is available from the New Zealand Nurses Organisation (2005) and the College of Nurses Aotearoa (2005). A sample portfolio template is available from the New Zealand Nurses Organisation (2005). It is also recommended that you read a text that addresses portfolio development, listed in the 'Recommended reading' (Andre & Heartfield 2006). Always ensure that your portfolio contains the relevant evidence to meet the continuing competency requirements for renewal of your registration.

Defining competence

It is essential for you to fully understand the competency standards, as you will be assessed according to these standards. To do so, you will need to understand the meaning of the terms competence and competent. **Competence** is 'the combination of skills, knowledge, attitudes, values and abilities that underpin effective performance as a nurse' (Nursing Council of New Zealand 2008c). **Competent** means 'the person has competence across all the domains of competencies applicable to the . . . nurse, at a standard that is judged to be appropriate for the level of nurse being assessed' (Nursing Council of New Zealand 2007b p 20).

It is very important to note that competence is not simply 'doing' a skill, or 'getting the work done', and it includes your skills, knowledge, attitudes, values and abilities. To be considered competent, you will need to demonstrate your competence in *all* the domains or aspects of nursing practice. The Nursing Council of New Zealand specifically states that a nurse must be competent when assessed against all of the competencies (Nursing Council of New Zealand 2008d). (The assessment of competence during clinical placement will be addressed in detail in Ch 13.)

Cultural competence

Cultural safety is a very important concept in New Zealand nursing practice, and is a core competency for all nurses (Nursing Council of New Zealand 2007a p 7, 2007b p 9). Cultural safety is defined as:

> . . . the effective nursing practice of a person from another culture, and is determined by that person or family [and requires that] the nurse delivering the nursing service will have undertaken a process of reflection on his or her own cultural identity and will recognise [its] impact . . . on professional practice (Nursing Council of New Zealand 2005 p 7).

In addition, all nurses are expected to apply the principles of the **Treaty of Waitangi** or Te Tiriti o Waitangi to their nursing practice as part of meeting competency standards for practice (Nursing Council of New Zealand 2007a p 6, 2007b p 7). (Ch 6 specifically addresses these concepts in New Zealand nursing practice.)

It is important for nurses in New Zealand to understand the issues associated with culture and ethnicity and their impact on health, and it is highly recommended that you read about these concepts in the source listed in the 'Recommended reading' (Dowd et al 2009), as well as studying Chapter 6 in detail.

Structure of the competencies

The competencies for registered nurses and nurse assistants/enrolled nurses are structured according to four **domains** that are major aspects, areas or parameters of nursing practice. Within each domain are a number of **competencies** that are defined areas of skilled performance. Each competency has a number of **indicators** that serve as examples of the competency. Tables 5.7 and 5.8 outline the key aspects of each domain.

QUESTION FOR REFLECTION

How do the competencies for nurses compare to the competency standards for nurses in your country?

TABLE 5.7 Competencies for Registered Nurses in New Zealand: overview of the domains

Domain	Key aspects (reflected by the competencies and indicators)
1. Professional responsibility	Professional, legal, ethical responsibilities Knowledge base (for safe practice) Judgment Accountability for supervision and delegation Recognition of own scope of practice/limitations Understanding/application of principles of Treaty of Waitangi or Te Tiriti o Waitangi Abiding by legislation Ensuring cultural safety Maintaining safety and security
2. Management of nursing care	Use of the nursing process: assessment, planning, implementation and evaluation of nursing care (including competent therapeutic skills performance) Documentation Confidentiality Education, information and advocacy Management of emergencies Reflective practice Professional development
Alternatives to Domain 2 competencies for nurses practising in management, education, policy and research	Promotion of an environment conducive to the demonstration and evaluation of the competencies Promotion of an environment that enables safe, effective, ethical nursing Integration of evidence-based theory and best practice into education Promotion and utilisation of research Professional development

TABLE 5.7 Competencies for Registered Nurses in New Zealand: overview of the domains—*cont'd*

Domain	Key aspects (reflected by the competencies and indicators)
3. Interpersonal relationships	Therapeutic relationship management Negotiation of partnership with clients/family Information/education Advocacy Communication with clients and healthcare team Confidentiality
Alternatives to Domain 3 competencies for nurses practising in management, education, policy and research	Interpersonal relationship management Communicates effectively with members of the healthcare team
4. Interprofessional healthcare and quality improvement	Communication, collaboration and participation within healthcare team Coordination and management of care Quality improvement

Source: Nursing Council of New Zealand 2007b.

TABLE 5.8 Competencies for Nurse Assistants and Enrolled Nurses in New Zealand: overview of the domains

Domain	Key aspects (reflected by the competencies and indicators)
1. Professional responsibility	Professional, legal, ethical responsibilities Understanding/application of principles of Treaty of Waitangi or Te Tiriti o Waitangi Recognition of own scope of practice and registered nurse scope of practice Safety and security Accountability and responsibility Dignity and respect Cultural safety Professional development
2. Management of care	Care provision under registered nurse supervision (including competent therapeutic skills performance) Practises within own scope of practice Time management Data gathering and reporting Documentation
3. Interpersonal relationships	Effective communication with clients
4. Interprofessional healthcare and quality improvement	Communication and collaboration with healthcare team Evaluation/reporting to registered nurse

Source: Nursing Council of New Zealand 2007a.

Required resources

You will need to obtain copies of the documents listed in Table 5.9.

TABLE 5.9 Resources for overseas nurses and international nursing students in New Zealand

Student/nurse	Document	Source
All nursing students and nurses	Code of Conduct for Nurses, March 2008	www.nursingcouncil.org.nz/code%20of%20conduct%20March%202008.pdf
	Guidelines for Cultural Safety, the Treaty of Waitangi and Māori Health in Nursing Education and Practice, March 2005	www.nursingcouncil.org.nz/Cultural%20Safety.pdf
Bachelor of Nursing students Registered nurses	Competencies for Registered Nurses, December 2007	www.nursingcouncil.org.nz/NA%20Comps%20final.pdf
	Competencies for Nurse Assistants and Enrolled Nurses, December 2007	www.nursingcouncil.org.nz/NA%20Comps%20final.pdf
Registered nurses Nurse educators, managers, researchers, leaders	Competencies for Registered Nurses, December 2007	www.nursingcouncil.org.nz/NA%20Comps%20final.pdf
	Competence Assessment Form for the Registered Nurse Scope of Practice, 2006	www.nursingcouncil.org.nz/Competence%20assessment%20form%20 for%20RN%20June%2006.pdf
	Competence Assessment Form for the Nurse Assistant and the Enrolled Nurse Scopes of Practice, 2006	www.nursingcouncil.org.nz/Competence%20assessment%20form%20 for%20NA%20EN%20June%2006.pdf
Certificate for Nurse Assistants/Certificate in Nursing students Nurse assistants/enrolled nurses	Competencies for Nurse Assistants and Enrolled Nurses, December 2007	www.nursingcouncil.org.nz/NA%20Comps%20final.pdf

CHAPTER HIGHLIGHTS

- Legislation requires nurses to meet professional standards and be competent.
- Nursing regulatory authorities have developed regulatory frameworks to ensure that nurses seeking registration meet professional standards and competencies.
- Nurses are expected to maintain portfolios containing evidence of their continuing competence.
- Codes of ethics outline the morals and values nurses are expected to have.
- Codes of conduct and codes of professional conduct outline the behavioural standards and expectations of nurses.
- Competency standards specify the expected core competencies, which nurses—and nursing students—must meet in their practice.

- Competence is a broad concept that includes skills, knowledge, attitudes, values and abilities—and is not limited to the performance of clinical skills.
- To be considered competent, nurses must meet *all* of the relevant competency standards.
- To be considered competent, all nurses must demonstrate sound English language skills.
- To be considered competent, nurses in New Zealand must be able to demonstrate cultural safety and the application of the principles of the Treaty of Waitangi in their practice.

Self-test questions

Plain numbered questions are for all readers; 'a' questions are for readers in Australia; 'b' questions are for readers in New Zealand.

1a. Obtain, read and summarise the relevant documents listed in Table 5.5.

1b. Obtain, read and summarise the relevant documents listed in Table 5.9.

2. What is the name of the law that governs the practice of nurses where you are working or studying?

3. What organisation has developed the standards and competencies where you are working or studying?

4. Describe the nursing regulatory framework where you are working or studying, with respect to nursing standards and competencies.

5. State the purpose of the codes of ethics and/or conduct where you are working or studying.

6. Describe the purpose of the nursing competencies or competency standards where you are working or studying.

7. Outline the structure of the nursing competencies or competency standards where you are working or studying.

8. Discuss in detail the meaning of the terms 'competence' and 'competent', and provide clinical nursing examples of each.

9a. Using the set of national competency standards most applicable to you, provide an example of competent practice (from your own clinical practice if possible) for *each* of the competency units.

9b. Using the competencies for the scope of practice most applicable to you, provide an example of competent practice (from your own clinical practice if possible) for *each* of the competencies.

10a. Read and summarise a recent journal article about nursing competency standards in Australia using the 'Article summary sheet' (R1) on the CD Part 3—Reader resources.

10b. Read and summarise a recent journal article about nursing competency standards in New Zealand using the 'Article summary sheet' (R1) on the CD Part 3—Reader resources.

11. Review the key terms and any other new vocabulary, terms and abbreviations from this chapter, and then update your 'Language list' (R2) on the CD Part 3—Reader resources.

12. Answer the 'Learning objectives' at the start of this chapter as if they were examination questions.

References

Australian Nursing and Midwifery Council 2002a Code of Ethics for Nurses in Australia. Online. Available www.anmc.org.au/docs/ANMC_Code_of_Ethics.pdf 23 Oct 2007

Australian Nursing and Midwifery Council 2002b National Competency Standards for the Enrolled Nurse. Online. Available www.anmc.org.au/docs/Publications/Competency%20 standards%20EN.pdf 23 Oct 2007

Australian Nursing and Midwifery Council 2002c Principles for the assessment of National Competency Standards. Online. Available www.anmc.org.au/docs/Principles%20for%20 the%20Assessment.pdf 23 Oct 2007

Australian Nursing and Midwifery Council 2003 Code of Professional Conduct for Nurses in Australia. Online. Available www.anmc.org.au/docs/ANMC_Professional_Conduct.pdf 23 Oct 2007

Australian Nursing and Midwifery Council 2006 National Competency Standards for the Registered Nurse. Online. Available www.anmc.org.au/docs/Competency_standards_ RN.pdf 23 Oct 2007

Australian Nursing and Midwifery Council 2008a Development of a national framework for the demonstration of continuing competence for nurses and midwives. Online. Available www.anmc.org.au/projects/current_projects.php#continuingcompetence 27 July 2008

Australian Nursing and Midwifery Council 2008b National Continuing Competence Framework (Draft 3). Online. Available www.anmc.org.au/docs/Research%20and%20 Policy/Continuing%20Competencies/Draft%203%20CC%20Framework.pdf 27 July 2008

Australian Nursing Federation 2008 Continuing professional education online. Online. Available www.onwebfast.com/anf/pd_record_demo.htm 6 Mar 2008

College of Nurses Aotearoa 2005 Competence to practice and professional portfolios. Online. Available www.nurse.org.nz/guidelines/gl_portfolio.htm 6 Mar 2008

Council of Australian Governments 2008a Council of Australian Governments' Communique, 26 March 2008. Online. Available www.coag.gov.au/meetings/ 130407/ 12 May 2008

Council of Australian Governments 2008b Intergovernmental agreement for a national registration and accreditation scheme for the health professions,

Online. Available www.coag.gov.au/meetings/260308/docs/iga_health_workforce.rtf / 12 May 2008

New Zealand Nurses Organisation 2005 Professional portfolios. Online. Available www.nzno.org.nz/Site/Resources/Portfolios.aspx 7 Mar 2008

New Zealand Ministry of Health 2006 Health Practitioners Competence Assurance Act 2003. Online. Available www.moh.govt.nz/hpca 12 May 2007

Nurses and Midwives Board of Western Australia 2007 Professional competence. Online. Available www.nmbwa.org.au/1/1119/50/professional_co.pm 7 Mar 2008

Nursing Council of New Zealand 2005 Guidelines for Cultural Safety, the Treaty of Waitangi and Māori Health in Nursing Education and Practice. Online. Available www. nursingcouncil.org.nz/Cultural%20Safety.pdf 14 May 2008

Nursing Council of New Zealand 2006a Competence Assessment Form for the Nurse Assistant and the Enrolled Nurse Scopes of Practice. Online. Available www. nursingcouncil.org.nz/Competence%20assessment%20form%20for%20NA%20EN%20 June%2006.pdf 14 May 2008

Nursing Council of New Zealand 2006b Competence Assessment Form for the Registered Nurse Scope of Practice. Online. Available www.nursingcouncil.org.nz/Competence%20 assessment%20form%20for%20RN%20June%2006.pdf 14 May 2008

Nursing Council of New Zealand 2007a Competencies for Nurse Assistants and Enrolled Nurses. Online. Available www.nursingcouncil.org.nz/NA%20Comps%20final.pdf 14 May 2008

Nursing Council of New Zealand 2007b Competencies for Registered Nurses. Online. Available www.nursingcouncil.org.nz/RN%20Comps%20final.pdf 14 May 2008
Nursing Council of New Zealand 2008a Code of Conduct for Nurses. Online. Available www.nursingcouncil.org.nz/code%20of%20conduct%20March%202008.pdf 14 May 2008
Nursing Council of New Zealand 2008b Continuing Competence Framework. Online. Available www.nursingcouncil.org.nz/contcomp.html 14 May 2008
Nursing Council of New Zealand 2008c Definition of competence. Online. Available www.nursingcouncil.org.nz/contcomp.html#DefComp 14 May 2008
Nursing Council of New Zealand 2008d Recertification programme (audit) requirements. Online. Available www.nursingcouncil.org.nz/contcomp.html#Comps 14 May 2008

Recommended reading

Andre K, Heartfield K 2006 Nursing portfolios: evidence for professional practice. Elsevier, Sydney
Dowd T, Eckermann K, Jeffs L 2009 Culture and ethnicity. In: Crisp J, Taylor C (eds) Potter & Perry's fundamentals of nursing, 3rd edn. Elsevier, Sydney, Ch 8
Walton, J, Marriott R 2008 Culturally competent care. In: Brown D, Edwards H (eds) Lewis's medical–surgical nursing: assessment and management of clinical problems, 2nd edn. Elsevier, Sydney, pp 22–34

CHAPTER 6

Cultural safety in New Zealand nursing practice

By Gill Scrymgeour[1]

'There is much we could learn from New Zealand nurses about cultural safety . . . it is so much more than cultural awareness and cultural sensitivity. Cultural competence seems to be a most appropriate concept for nurses in Australian too.'

Gabrielle, Australia

CHAPTER OUTLINE

Learning objectives
Key terms
Defining culture
About New Zealand
Nursing in New Zealand
The Treaty of Waitangi
Biculturalism
Cultural safety
  Cultural safety practices for Māori
  Personal reflections on cultural safety
Chapter highlights
Self-test questions
References

LEARNING OBJECTIVES

1. Gain an insight into the history that shapes nursing practice in New Zealand.
2. Understand the meaning and importance of biculturalism.
3. Understand the importance of cultural safety in New Zealand nursing practice.
4. Be aware of the traditions and customary practices important to Māori that impact on their physical, emotional and spiritual wellbeing.

1 The author gratefully acknowledges the contribution of Kathy Monson for her support and Di Wepa who provided encouragement, guidance and critique for authenticity of Māori content.

5. Be able to articulate how nurses in New Zealand honour the Treaty of Waitangi within their nursing practice.

Key terms (are in bold in the text)

ahutanga Māori (Māori tradition)
aroha (love)
biculturalism
competencies for nurses (formerly called competencies for scopes of practice)
cultural safety (kawa whakaruruhau)
domains (of competencies)
dysconsciousness
iwi (tribe)
karakia (prayers)
karanga (call of welcome)
kaumatua (male Māori elder)
kaupapa (process of Māori custom)
kawa (ritual of Māori custom)
kawa whakaruruhau (cultural safety)
kuia (female Māori elder)
Māori
marae (Māori settlement)
mihi (informal speech)
noa (safe)
Pakeha (non-Māori New Zealander)
participation
partnership
protection
reflect
powhiri (welcome ceremony)
Tangata Whenua (Indigenous people)
tangi (funeral)
tangihanga (funeral ceremony)
taonga (treasures)
tapu (sacred or 'off limits')
tikanga Māori (Māori custom)
Tiriti o Waitangi (Treaty of Waitangi)
tohunga (spiritual leader)
Treaty of Waitangi
tuku wairua (ceremony for the dying)
waiata (song)
wairua (spirit)
whaikorero (formal)
whakahoki (response to karanga)
whanau (family)

This chapter provides a summary of the history of **cultural safety (kawa whakaruruhau)** within the nursing framework, and outlines the cultural safety practices expected of nurses in New Zealand. The incorporation of this concept into the competency standards for nurses within the **competencies for nurses (formerly called competencies for scopes of practice)** established by the Nursing Council of New Zealand are discussed. It also provides explanations and meanings that will assist in implementing cultural safety for **Māori** clients into practice.

Defining culture

Our way of living is our culture. It is our taken-for-grantedness that determines and defines our culture. The way we brush our teeth, the way we bury people, the way we express ourselves through our art, religion, eating habits, rituals, humour, science, law and sport, and the way we celebrate occasions (such as twenty-first birthdays or weddings) is our culture. All these actions we carry out consciously and unconsciously (Wepa 2005 p 31).

About New Zealand

In the past, the vast majority of people in other countries did not know of New Zealand or where it was located. Many would think of its location as being 'somewhere near Australia'. New Zealand today has a much higher profile internationally. It has become recognised as a strong sporting nation with internationally renowned teams such as the rugby 'All Blacks', the cricket 'Black Caps' and the netball 'Silver Ferns'. New Zealand's home-grown movie producer, Peter Jackson, and his *Lord of the Rings* trilogy allowed millions of people from around the world to take a peak at this beautiful country through his stunning cinematography. Many have now discovered this 'Land of the Long White Cloud—Aotearoa'.

Nursing in New Zealand

Nurses educated in New Zealand are well respected internationally for their high standards and ability to adapt and work in most healthcare institutes around the world. Nursing is viewed as a mobile profession with thousands of nurses migrating to New Zealand each year in search of better pay, working conditions or improved lifestyle opportunities.

They may have noticed on arriving that New Zealand is not just an English-speaking Western country, but is actually a bicultural nation with two recognised languages (Māori and English), and its own unique culture and traditions. For many, the journey of discovery and the realisation of what it means to practise in a culturally safe manner, which is unique to New Zealand, takes time.

Sometimes, the lack of knowledge about New Zealand's cultural context can be interpreted as racism or cultural insensitivity. This could also be viewed as a form of 'dysconscious racism' (Papps, personal communication, 2007), which is a concept created by Joyce King in 1990 in her seminal work (cited in Brandon 2007). **Dysconsciousness** is an impaired way of thinking, often using generalist assumptions based on distorted views of reality, history and oneself in relation to other cultures. King views this impaired way of thinking more as a result of miseducation.

The Treaty of Waitangi

In order to understand the concept of **biculturalism** and cultural safety, it is first important to understand the history of New Zealand. The first settlers travelled by outrigger canoe from Polynesia in approximately 1200–1300 AD. These inhabitants were the ancestors of Māori. Abel Tasman was the first European to visit and trade with Māori. Captain Cook stepped ashore in 1773. The first British missionaries arrived in 1814. In 1935, the Declaration of Independence was signed recognising Aotearoa New Zealand as a sovereign nation under the leadership of Rangatira (Chiefdom) (McKinney & Smith 2005).

The **Treaty of Waitangi (Tiriti o Waitangi)** was signed on 6 February 1840. It was an agreement between Māori and the Crown (Britain). It is considered to be the founding document of New Zealand (Durie 1998). The Treaty recognised Māori as Indigenous people (**Tangata Whenua**) of the land and guaranteed protection of their customary rights by the Crown. In return, Māori agreed to the Crown providing governorship to the land. According to the Māori version of the Treaty, this did not include sovereignty, whereas the English version did (McKinney & Smith 2005). The interpretation of the Treaty has created debate. Māori believe that their rights have not been protected and this is evident in the disparity of health status between Māori and non-Māori New Zealanders (**Pakeha**) (Ministry of Health 2002b, Papps 2002).

In 1975, the Waitangi Tribunal was formed, and continues to this day, to work towards addressing some of the injustices for Māori created by the Crown (the government) since the signing of the Treaty. The Tribunal emphasises that it is the prinvciples of the Treaty document that are important and not the debate over the literal translations. This enables the Treaty (principles) to be applied to situations that were not foreseen at the signing of the Treaty of Waitangi (State Services Commission 2005). Key principles that are considered within the healthcare arena are **partnership**, **protection** and **participation** (Ministry of Health 2002a p 2), often referred to as 'the 3 Ps'.

Partnership within a healthcare setting is honouring the ongoing relationship between the Crown and **iwi** (tribe) (Article One, Treaty of Waitangi). This includes agents of the Crown such as District Health Boards and other government organisations. For a nurse working in New Zealand, this will include developing a therapeutic relationship with the client/patient, respecting cultural differences, discussing options and involving them in the decisions about their care.

Protection refers to the obligations of the Crown to protect Māori interests, treasures (**taonga**) and property (Article Two, Treaty of Waitangi). Within a healthcare setting, this extends to obligations of the government to provide funding for Māori health initiatives. In practice, this involves protecting their physical, spiritual, emotional, mental and family health.

Participation incorporates Royal protection (i.e. the rights and privileges accorded to British subjects) (Article Three, Treaty of Waitangi), and calls for positive Māori involvement at the highest levels of decision making and within all aspects of society. This includes an expectation that Māori will be enabled to participate in the consultation process in healthcare planning. Such an approach also acknowledges the '4 Ms model', which refers to Māori Management of Matters Māori (Wepa, personal communication, 2007) and recognition of a bicultural society. As a nurse, it is important to consult and involve the client/patient in all decisions. This includes recognition that health issues may extend to **whanau** (family) and **iwi** (tribe), but only after discussion and obtaining consent from the client.

Biculturalism

At thc same time the Waitangi Tribunal was established, the concept of biculturalism was also gaining momentum and became a basis for policies to improve opportunities for Māori. By 1985, it was being promoted within the healthcare system. The essence of biculturalism was that it was the recognition of two distinct cultures—Māori and Pakeha—that coexisted within New Zealand society. Ideally, this extended to sharing control of decision making and resources (Durie 1998). In reality, this was not always evident and the definition often became blurred. Durie regarded biculturalism as a continuum of goals and structural arrangements, which are still in the process of being realised. This continuum ranges from a monocultural mainstream institution at one extreme to an independent Māori organisation at the other.

Many healthcare institutions still continue to practise within the middle-range of this continuum. For these institutions, there remains an emphasis on cultural enrichment of staff and cultural sensitivity to Māori protocol, rather than addressing the fundamental issues of the Treaty's promise to allow full participation and partnership in decision making and policy development (Durie 1998). Many worthwhile initiatives have been introduced that go beyond basic cultural sensitivity and work towards true biculturalism.

Under the *Public Health and Disability Act* 2000, health professionals in New Zealand are obligated to recognise and respect the Treaty of Waitangi. This Act sets down statutory obligations of the District Health Boards (DHBs) to improve the health outcomes for Māori (Ministry of Health 2005). DHBs must allow for Māori to have greater contribution in decision making and participation in the delivery of health and disability services to Māori. The concept of 'by Māori for Māori' (the '4 Ms model') has become fundamental to many new Māori-led initiatives, which are working successfully in parallel to mainstream developments (Wilson & Roberts 2005).

Cultural safety

The concept of **kawa whakarurhau** or **cultural safety** within nursing practice was first introduced by Irihapeti Ramsden in the 1980s. This concept was later endorsed by the Nursing Council of New Zealand who initiated a set of guidelines for the teaching of cultural safety to nursing students. By 1992, the Nursing Council also required that 20% of the content of their state nursing examinations related to cultural safety (Clarke 2005).

Cultural safety in New Zealand was often viewed as a Māori issue only. This was redressed in 2002 through the results of audits of nursing curricula and consultation with Ramsden who had now become the educational consultant for cultural safety for the Nursing Council. It was acknowledged that the teaching of cultural safety, the Treaty of Waitangi and Māori health issues needed to be separated out and taught with clear learning outcomes in order to improve health outcomes for Māori, as well as other minority groups in New Zealand (Clarke 2005). The Nursing Council's revised definition in 2005 stated:

> Cultural safety is the effective nursing or midwifery practice of a person or family from another culture, and is determined by that person or family. Culture includes, but is not restricted to age or generation; gender; sexual orientation; occupation and socioeconomic status; ethnic origin or migrant experience; religious or spiritual belief; and disability.
>
> The nurse or midwife delivering the nursing or midwifery service will have undertaken a process of reflection on his or her own cultural identity and will recognise the impact that his or her personal culture has on professional practice. Unsafe cultural practice comprises any action that diminishes, demeans or disempowers the cultural identity and wellbeing of an individual (Nursing Council of New Zealand 2005 p 7).

Papps succinctly states 'the essence of cultural safety is personal identification of attitudes that an individual may have towards a person or a group of people who may be different from the nurse' (2002 p 96).

The key to either definition is in the nurse's ability to **reflect** on his or her own attitudes to differences in an individual. It is also important to note that it is the client—and not the nurse—who determines whether the nursing care is culturally safe.

It is a statutory requirement that nurses practising in New Zealand do so in a culturally safe manner and honour the Treaty of Waitangi. All nurses in New Zealand are assessed against the four **domains** contained in the Nursing Council's **competencies for nurses** for their competency-based annual practising certificate.

This set of competencies includes specific reference to the Treaty and to cultural safety. Competency 1.2 states that it is essential that the nurse 'demonstrates the ability to apply the principles of the Treaty of Waitangi/Te Tiriti O Waitangi [i.e. Tiriti o Waitangi] to nursing practice' (Nursing Council of New Zealand 2007 p 7). Competency 1.5 specifically deals with cultural safety for all clients and is not restricted solely to the care of Māori clients. It states that nurses are expected to practise 'in a manner that the client determines as being culturally safe' (p 9).

?

QUESTION FOR REFLECTION

Reflect on your own cultural values and traditions. What key values currently guide your nursing practice?

Cultural safety practices for Māori

One way to improve the health status of Māori is through a culturally aware workforce. Cultural safety is about respecting difference and this is where this concept and honouring the Treaty of Waitangi merge for nurses working in a healthcare facility in New Zealand. Māori have their own distinct beliefs about keeping themselves free from harm physically, emotionally and spiritually. This is particularly evident in Māori tradition (**ahutanga Māori**) and Māori custom (**tikanga Māori**).

Tikanga Māori is a form of social etiquette/control. It deals with right and wrong and therefore focuses on the correct way of doing something. Many Māori embrace tikanga Māori as a set of guiding principles that empower them and that they are bound to uphold. Mead (2003 p 7) suggests that it can be described as 'Māori philosophy in practice and as the practical force of Māori'. It is important to be aware that Māori tradition and customary practices may differ from one tribe (**iwi**) to another. There is often a ritual aspect to tikanga Māori; some Māori still believe that if this ritual is carried out incorrectly or broken, misfortune will occur as punishment from Māori gods. The male (**kaumatua**) and female (**kuia**) elders are expected to be conversant with tikanga.

Sometimes, breaches of tikanga may be met with anger, scolding and even abuse. One example of this is when visitors visit a ceremonial meeting house within a Māori settlement (**marae**) and do not follow correct protocol. Although the recipient of this may feel mortified at this reaction, the practice is considered a necessary and sharp lesson in order to inform them of their mistake (Mead 2003).

One time when ritual is very important is during and following the death of a Māori client. When a Māori client is dying, a special ceremony (**tuku wairua**) is carried out by either a minister of the church or spiritual leader (**tohunga**). It is similar to the last rites within some religions. It is a releasing of the spirit (**wairua**) and asking it to leave. Just prior to this happening, the family members usually start arriving in large numbers to keep vigil and provide support. Prayers (**karakia**) are performed, and the elders normally address the dying person. Once the person has died, it is believed that the wairua leaves the body, but does not go far away. Many Māori also believe that the wairua watches the funeral ceremony (**tangihanga**). Mead (2003) suggests this is why orators at the **tangi** speak in loud voices when they address the dead, usually stressing the good things about that person. They will also request that the wairua depart often to the land of their forebears, Hawaiki-nui.

Nurses working within the community, in particular, need to be aware of the process (**kaupapa**) and ritual (**kawa**) of tikanga Māori. The opportunity will no doubt arise to be part of a welcome ceremony (**powhiri**) or a visit to the local marae and maybe even to attend a tangi.

Each marae has its own set of protocols. Visitors are expected to wait at the entrance until they receive a call of welcome (**karanga**), which is performed by a kuia. It is an invitation to come in peace and love (**aroha**). If the visitors are not Māori, a Māori guide who goes before them replies with a form of acknowledgment (**whakahoki**). Following this, the visitor will be welcomed and a powhiri will occur, which involves much speech making—some formal (**whaikorero**) and some informal (**mihi**)—and plenty of singing (**waiata**) and prayers. All of this is carried out in the Māori language. Sometimes, you may be lucky to have a guide who will translate for you, but often there is an expectation that you should understand what is being said.

A powhiri also occurs in many situations outside of the marae. This may include welcoming a Māori staff member into an organisation or new students into a New Zealand tertiary institute and therefore is a process worth being familiar with.

Tikanga Māori is also evident in the Māori concept of something that is sacred or off limits (**tapu**) or is considered safe (**noa**) (Durie 1998). Historically, Māori society was communal and these sets of practical rules/values were designed to protect and maintain a healthy community. This regulatory system allowed people within a community to clearly know what was off limits to them and what was safe. For this reason, tapu and noa are not always static but are dynamic and change according to circumstance (Durie 1998). Therefore, something that was off limits or tapu could be replaced with noa, rendering the original situation to be safe again.

One common example of this is when a patient dies. The room the person died in would become tapu and could not be used. This tapu would only be lifted to noa once the room was cleaned and blessed. This is one example of a customary practice that is also a widely used public health and hygiene practice. In many healthcare institutes, this tapu extends to the elevators in which the deceased are transported. No food must be taken into that particular lift. This author received the admonishment and wrath from a member of the public when she unwittingly carried her lunch into one of these designated lifts—a sharp and memorable lesson learnt! It is wise to check the notices on hospital lifts before walking in with your meal.

Table 6.1 provides examples of common tapu situations that the nurse may encounter. In striving for cultural safety, there is a risk of falling into the trap of stereotyping individuals. Many Māori look European and assuming a client is not Māori can become a culturally harmful situation to the client or the nurse. Some Māori prefer to accept their European traditions over Māori and assuming a 'one size fits all' approach to your client is a good example of dysconscious racism. The best advice is to develop a rapport with your client first, ask questions and respect their point of view and requests.

It is not the objective to include all examples of tikanga Māori or a complete list of situations that may be considered tapu in this chapter. You need to consider this an

TABLE 6.1 Common tapu situations

Part of body	Beliefs and practices
Head	The head is a sacred part of the body. Ask permission to touch someone's head. Do not pass food over someone's head. Do not step over someone lying down. Do not burn or throw away hair; put it in a tissue and allow the patient to discard it. Use separate towels and face cloths for the face and head. Head pillows should not be used to sit on or for under the legs.
Blood and body parts	Do not discard placenta (whenua), as it is considered part of the life blood of the family, and the family may wish to take it home and bury it in a special place back with the 'earth mother'. All body parts are to be offered back to the client (even following laboratory testing). Wrap nail clippings into a tissue and offer them back to the client to dispose of. Menstruating women are tapu; they must not go into the sea (to gather seafood), garden or ride horses.
Food	Do not put hats, combs or hairbrushes on the kitchen table. Do not wash clothes, babies or their nappies in a kitchen sink. Do not sit on any table or bench on which food may be prepared or served. Do not put bedpans, urinals or wash bowls on the bedside table from which the patient may eat. Do not store blood, body parts or specimens in the same fridge as food.

introduction only and it is highly recommended that you read the complete sources referenced in this chapter.

?

QUESTION FOR REFLECTION

What actions or behaviours would be considered tapu in your country? Are these similar to tikanga Māori?

Personal reflections on cultural safety

In order to appreciate and respect cultural difference, you must first acknowledge your own history and culture. I am a Pakeha. Although born in New Zealand, I moved to Sri Lanka with my parents when still a baby. During my childhood and early adolescence, I lived and went to school in India and Pakistan. I learnt to live among and respect the traditions and cultural rules of the countries in which I lived. I needed always to be mindful, however, that I was a visitor and felt privileged to experience first hand the rich history and culture of those countries.

When I moved back to New Zealand, I began to appreciate the richness of our New Zealand culture. I did not know very much about tikanga Māori—the learning did not happen overnight and still continues. As a registered nurse in New Zealand, I know that it is my responsibility to become informed and responsive to all cultural and ethnic groups. I am also aware of the importance of improving health outcomes for Māori and work towards this objective within my nursing practice. This too will be expected of you if you choose to work in New Zealand.

CHAPTER HIGHLIGHTS

- New Zealand is a bicultural nation with its own unique culture and traditions.
- The Treaty of Waitangi/Tiriti o Waitangi is the founding document of New Zealand.
- The Treaty recognises Māori as the Tangata Whenua of the land and guarantees their protection by the Crown.
- Māori believe their rights have not been protected and this is evident in the disparity between the health status of Māori and Pakeha.
- Under the *Public Health and Disability Act* 2000, New Zealand health professionals are obligated to recognise and respect the Treaty of Waitangi.
- Three guiding principles of the Treaty within healthcare are partnership, protection and participation.
- The concept of cultural safety within nursing practice in New Zealand was first introduced in the 1980s and is included in the Nursing Council's competencies.
- Cultural safety is about identifying personal attitudes to an individual who may be different from the nurse.
- It is the client who determines whether the nursing care is culturally safe.
- Nurses need to be aware of the importance of process and ritual of tikanga Māori.
- Māori have their own beliefs about keeping themselves free from harm physically, emotionally and spiritually.
- Early Māori society was communal and sets of practical rules/values such as tapu and noa were implemented to protect and maintain a healthy community.
- A registered nurse in New Zealand is responsible for improving the health outcomes for Māori, as well as being informed and responsive to all cultural and ethnic groups.

Self-test questions

1. You are asked the following question in a job interview or during your clinical placement: 'How will you implement the principles of the Treaty of Waitangi into your nursing practice?' How would you answer this?
2. Consider your own cultural background and practices. Would any of these need to be acknowledged and perhaps adapted in order to practise in a culturally safe manner in New Zealand?
3. When planning and implementing nursing care for your Māori client, what 'tapu' considerations first need to be identified in order not to offend?
4. When caring for a Māori client who has died, what key cultural safety practices do you need to be aware of? (You may need to refer to your local healthcare institution's policy and procedure guidelines to answer this question completely.)
5. Review the key terms and any other new vocabulary, terms and abbreviations from this chapter, and then update your 'Language list' (R2) on the CD Part 3—Reader resources.
6. Answer the 'Learning objectives' at the start of this chapter as if they were examination questions.

References

Brandon L 2007 On dysconsciousness: an interview with Joyce E King. Online. Available www.leaonline.com/doi/pdfplus/10.1207/s15326993es4002_12 20 Sept 2007

Clarke M 2005 Preface. In: Wepa D (ed) Cultural safety in Aotearoa New Zealand. Pearson Prentice-Hall, Auckland, pp v–vii

Durie M 1998 Whaiora: Māori health development, 2nd edn. Oxford University Press, Auckland

McKinney C, Smith N 2005 Te Tiriti o Waitangi or the Treaty of Waitangi: What is the difference? In: Wepa D (ed) Cultural safety in Aotearoa New Zealand. Pearson Prentice-Hall, Auckland

Mead H M 2003 Tikanga Māori: living by Māori values. Huia Publishing, Wellington

Ministry of Health 2002a He Korowai Oranga: Māori health strategy. Online. Available www.moh.govt.nz/moh.nsf/pagesma/304/$File/he-korowai-oranga-english.pdf 20 Sept 2007

Ministry of Health 2002b Reducing inequalities in health. Ministry of Health, Wellington

Ministry of Health 2005 The New Zealand Public Health and Disability Act 2000. Online. Available www.moh.govt.nz/moh.nsf/ea6005dc347e7bd44c2566a40079ae6f/e65f72c8749e91e74c2569620000b7ce?OpenDocument 20 Sept 2007

Nursing Council of New Zealand 2005 Guidelines for Cultural Safety, the Treaty of Waitangi and Māori Health in Nursing Education and Practice. Online. Available www.nursingcouncil.org.nz/Cultural%20Safety.pdf 29 Oct 2007

Nursing Council of New Zealand 2007 Competencies for Registered Nurses. Online. Available www.nursingcouncil.org.nz/RN%20Comps%20final.pdf 13 May 2008

Papps E 2002 Cultural safety: What is the question? In: Papps E (ed) Nursing in New Zealand: critical issues, different perspectives. Prentice Hall Health, Auckland, pp 95–107

State Services Commission 2005 All about the Treaty. Online. Available www.nzhistory.net.nz/files/documents/All_about_the_Treaty.pdf 24 Oct 2007

Wepa D 2005 Culture and ethnicity: What is the question? In: Wepa D (ed) Cultural safety in Aotearoa New Zealand. Pearson Prentice-Hall, Auckland, pp 30–8

Wilson D, Roberts M 2005 Māori health initiatives. In: Wepa D (ed) Cultural safety in Aotearoa New Zealand. Pearson Prentice-Hall, Auckland, pp 157–69

PART 3

The language of healthcare

CHAPTER 7

Overview of language in healthcare[2]

'It is like there are more languages in healthcare—not just English.'

Isabel, The Philippines

CHAPTER OUTLINE

LEARNING OBJECTIVE

1. Become familiar with the elements of language used in healthcare.

Key terms (are in bold in the text)

abbreviations	informal language
acronyms	jargon
colloquialisms	phrasal verbs
formal language	preposition
idioms	slang
informal idioms	terminology

An understanding of the elements of language assists the development of language skills. Knowing the part of speech or type of term, phrase or expression will assist you to learn informal language and jargon in healthcare.

2 The author gratefully acknowledges the contribution of Anita Gray for her assistance in providing resources to define the elements of language.

Formal and informal language

Formal and informal language is used in written and spoken English. The purpose, context and user determine the type of language used. **Formal language** is used for activities such as academic writing, business letters, written reports, speeches, oral presentations and formal discussion. In the healthcare setting, patient progress notes and referral letters would contain formal language. **Informal language** is used for personal letters, email messages and casual conversation.

Informal idioms

Idioms are defined as 'a number of words which, when taken together, have different meaning from the individual meanings of each word' (Seidl & McMordie 1988 pp 12–13). When idioms are used in informal language, they are often referred to as **colloquialisms**.

Phrasal verbs are **informal idioms** with a short verb and a **preposition**. **Slang** refers to the use of extremely informal idioms that are rarely used in written form, but are used in speech. 'Slang expressions relate to things that people feel strongly about (e.g. sex, family and emotional relationships, drink, drugs, conflict between social groups, work, physical and mental illness, death)' (Swan 1995 p 511). The use of slang could be limited to a particular culture or group. (See Ch 8 for further discussion and examples of informal idioms.)

Jargon

Jargon refers to the **terminology** related to a particular activity, occupation or profession, which is often meaningless to other people. For example, medical terminology is often difficult for people outside of the health professions to understand. **Abbreviations** are shortened forms of words, phrases or expressions, or the first initials of the words in a phrase or expression. Some of these types of abbreviations are used in the written form only and the full term is spoken, such as NCP for nursing care plan. **Acronyms** are a type of abbreviation, where the first initials of the words in a phrase or expression form a new word. Typically, an acronym forms a pronounceable word (Chabner 2005 p 311), such as NIDDM for non-insulin dependent diabetes mellitus. Others are written and pronounced by saying the names of the letters, such as ECG. (See Ch 9 for further discussion and examples of jargon.) Figure 7.1 describes the elements of language with examples for healthcare.

CHAPTER HIGHLIGHTS

- An understanding of the elements of language assists the development of language skills.
- Language is considered to be either formal or informal, and its uses vary according to the purpose, situation and user.
- Informal language is commonly used in healthcare, and includes idioms.

FIGURE 7.1 Overview of the types and elements of language

Formal language: used for academic writing, business letters, written reports, progress notes, referrals, speeches/oral presentations, formal discussion.

Informal language: used for personal letters, email messages, casual conversation.

Jargon: terminology related to a particular activity, occupation or profession, which is meaningless to other people (e.g. diaphoresis (sweating), oedema (swelling), bradycardia (slow pulse rate), epistaxis (blood nose)).
Can be formal or informal.

Idioms: a 'number of words which, when taken together, have different meaning from the individual meanings of each word' (Seidl & McMordie 1988 pp 12–13). Can be formal or informal.

Abbreviations (see Ch 9): shortened forms of words, terms or expressions.

Some are used in written and oral forms (e.g. stat (from statim) meaning immediately or now).

Some are written only (using the first initials of the words) and the full term is spoken (e.g. NCP for nursing care plan, which is pronounced nursing care plan).

Acronyms (see Ch 9): a type of abbreviation where a word is formed by using the first initial of the words of a phrase or expression.

Some acronyms are written and pronounced as a new word (e.g. NIDDM for non-insulin dependent diabetes, which is pronounced 'NIDDM').

Some acronyms are written and pronounced by saying the names of the letters (e.g. ECG for electrocardiogram, which is pronounced E-C-G).

Informal idioms

Colloquialisms (see Ch 8): informal idioms (e.g. 'fighting fit' means 'to be well' and 'running a temperature' means 'febrile').

Phrasal verbs (see Ch 8): informal idioms with a short verb and a preposition (e.g. 'come down with an illness' means 'to contract or develop an illness' and 'put up the IV fluid' means 'administer IV fluid via a flask').

Slang: very informal idioms; rarely written; used in speech; could be limited to a cultural group.

'Slang expressions relate to things that people feel strongly about (e.g. sex, family and emotional relationships, drink, drugs, conflict between social groups, work, physical and mental illness, death) (Swan 1995 p 511). For example, 'down the hatch' means 'to swallow' (e.g. medicine).

- Informal idioms are known as colloquialisms and, where a verb and preposition are used together, are called phrasal verbs.
- Jargon refers to the terminology related to an activity, occupation or profession.
- Abbreviations and acronyms (abbreviations using the initials of the words in a phrase) are a part of jargon.

Self-test questions

1. Write a brief definition and provide an example of the following terms: informal language; formal language; idiom; colloquialism; phrasal verb; slang; jargon; abbreviation; and acronym.
2. Update your 'Language list' (R2) on the CD Part 3—Reader resources.

References

Chabner D 2005 Medical terminology: a short course, 4th edn. Elsevier, St Louis
Seidl J, McMordie W 1988 English idioms, 5th edn. Oxford University Press, Oxford
Swan M 1995 Practical English usage. Oxford University Press, Oxford

CHAPTER 8

Informal language in healthcare[3]

By Anna Chur-Hansen, Taryn Elliott and M Bernadette Hally

'I am trying to talk with and listen to the local people, and watching local TV, so I can understand my patients better.'

Imran, Pakistan

CHAPTER OUTLINE

LEARNING OBJECTIVE

1. Become familiar with the informal language—colloquialisms and phrasal verbs—used in healthcare in Australia or New Zealand.

3 The authors gratefully acknowledge the contribution of Gill Scrymgeour in consulting about the New Zealand content of this chapter, and the work of Leticia Supple in the adaptation of Dr Anna Chur-Hansen's original work.

In Australia and New Zealand, informal language is used extensively. Patients and health professionals use colloquialisms and phrasal verbs. You will need to be familiar with these expressions to ensure excellent communication with your patients and colleagues.

Many of these expressions will probably seem strange to you. You do not need to use colloquialisms yourself, but it is very important that you understand what other people are saying to you. You will find that you need to be able to understand and use the phrasal verbs related to nursing care.

When you hear an unfamiliar expression, remember to ask the person who has said it, what the expression means (see Ch 2 for hints on developing your English and 'nursing English'). You could say: 'I am not familiar with that expression. Could you please repeat it?' or 'What does that expression mean?' If the person cannot explain the meaning to you, ask a teacher or colleague. You should write the new expression in the relevant section in this chapter, along with the meaning.

To hear how each expression is pronounced, listen to the CD Part 1—Audio, 'Pronunciation of colloquialisms' (A1) and 'Pronunciation of phrasal verbs' (A2).

The colloquialisms and phrasal verbs listed in this chapter are just some of the terms you will hear. Make sure you record other terms to expand your vocabulary.

Colloquialisms

By Anna Chur-Hansen and Taryn Elliott[4]

Colloquialisms could be used in general conversation, or in conversations directly related to health and healthcare. Some of the colloquialisms listed below are unique to Australia (Aus) or New Zealand (NZ), and this is noted in brackets beside the term or expression. Some colloquialisms used in Australia are specific to an area or state, so check with a local native speaker if you are unsure whether the term or expression is used where you live or work.

States of health or illness, including levels of energy

Tiredness

The following four sayings are all based on fairly vulgar meanings. Even so, they are commonly used in everyday speech, and might be used by the patient to a health professional.

I feel buggered.

I'm knackered.

I'm rooted.

I'm stuffed.

The following colloquialisms are fairly old-fashioned. You would probably hear them being used by older people.

I'm all tuckered out.

I'm done like a dog's dinner.

4 Adapted from Chur-Hansen (2005) and Chur-Hansen et al (2006).

I'm done in.

I'm dead beat.

Many people would use the following colloquialisms.

I'm bushed.

I've had it.

Feeling moderately well

When someone feels moderately well, they might use these sayings to their friends or to a health professional.

I'm fair to middling.

I'm so-so.

I'm feeling average.

Feeling well

Mostly older people would use the following sayings. 'Sweet as' is used by younger people.

I'm as fit as a fiddle.

I'm in tip-top shape.

I'm as fit as a mallee bull. (Aus)

I'm as fit as a box of fluffy ducks. (NZ)

I'm as good as gold.

I'm as sweet as. (NZ)

Feeling physically fit

Mostly older people would say these.

I'm as fit as a fiddle.

I'm in tip-top shape.

I'm as fit as a mallee bull. (Aus)

Feeling physically unfit

The following saying is used widely.

I am out of condition.

Appearing unwell

The following sayings would be used to describe someone who the speaker thought looked unwell or appeared anaemic. They would also be used if the observer thought that someone looked as if they had had a fright.

You look as pale as a ghost.

You are as white as a sheet.

Feeling physically unwell

The following sayings are both quite vulgar. You would not usually say them in polite company, but in certain circumstances a patient may say them to the doctor.

I feel shithouse. (Aus)

I feel like shit/crap.

The following sayings are used widely. Usually, the person would be referring to a physical ailment, but they could all theoretically refer to emotional and psychological states as well.

I feel crook.

I'm under the weather.

I'm not 100%.

I'm feeling ordinary.

I'm only 99%.

I'm feeling lousy.

I feel a bit off.

I am as sick as a dog.

I feel off colour.

I'm feeling wonky.

I'm feeling seedy.

I'm feeling woozy.

I've been feeling run down.

I am down and out.

I'm feeling iffy.

I'm stuffed.

I'm a bit wobbly.

I'm feeling dodgy. (Aus)

Quite often, when a person is unwell with a respiratory infection (commonly but incorrectly called 'flu') or gastric infection, or a non-specific illness, they will say that they have a 'wog'. If they are only sick for a day, they will say that it was a '24-hour wog' or 'bug'.

I've got a wog. (Aus)

There's a wog going around. (Aus)

I've got a 24-hour wog. (Aus)

I've got a lurgy.

I've got a lurg. (NZ)

I've got a bug.

There's a bug going around.

I've got a 24-hour bug.

Mentally unwell

The following are all common colloquialisms to describe someone who is perceived by the speaker as being mentally unwell. These terms would not ordinarily be used to describe your own state of mental health or illness, but rather to describe someone else's, either in conversation or to a healthcare professional.

He's not the full packet. (Aus)

He's not the full quid.

She's got a screw loose.

He's as mad as a meat axe.

He went bananas.

He's nuts.

He is around the bend.

He's as mad as a hatter.

She's gone ga-ga.

She's not the full cream. (NZ)

He's not playing with a full deck.

He's crazy.

She's loopy.

She's out of her tree.

He's out of his mind.

He has lost the plot. (Aus)

The following saying would be used mostly by older people.

She's as mad as a cut snake. (Aus)

Lacking in intellect

Obviously, all of the following terms are insulting and would usually be used to describe a third person or to someone's face if you wanted to be rude. 'Vegetable' or 'veggie' are especially rude terms used to refer to someone with a severe intellectual disability. A person with rural origins would be the most likely to call someone a 'galah', this being a parrot that is renowned in Australia for its silly behaviour.

She's a bit dim.

She's not a rocket scientist.

He's two snags short of a barbie. (Aus)

He's lost the plot.

She's hare-brained.

She's scatter-brained.

He's two bob short.

He's two bricks short of a load.

She's as thick as a brick.

She's as thick as a vegetable.

He's a veggie.

He's a bloody galah. (Aus)

The lights are on, but no one's home.

She's not the full quid. (Aus)

He's a wally.

He's as thick as two planks.

She's as dumb as dog shit. (Aus; vulgar)

She's a wacker. (Aus)

Additional colloquialisms

Emotions and emotional states

Happiness

Almost anyone might use the following sayings.

I'm over the moon.

I'm on top of the world.

I'm on cloud nine.

Usually, only younger people would say these.

I'm rapt.

I'm stoked.

Depression

Almost anyone might use these sayings.

I'm down in the dumps.

She's on a downer.

I am down.

I'm feeling blue.

She seemed as flat as a tack.

I feel flat.

Anger

Almost anyone from any age group could use the following sayings. They could use them to describe their own anger or someone else's.

I went berserk.

She screamed the place down.

She got upset and lost it.

All hell broke loose.

He is ropeable.

Mostly younger people would use these sayings.

He chucked a mental. (Aus)

He chucked a wobbly.

I'm spewing.

He has lost the plot.

She had a hissy fit.

Feeling unsettled (uneasy)

The following are used widely to describe a non-specific feeling of unease. They could refer to physical, mental or emotional health.

I feel out of sorts today.

I just don't feel right.

Regret

Mostly younger people would use these sayings.

What a bummer.

What a downer.

Bugger!

Damn!

Anxiety

The following saying might be used by any age group, but probably females would say this more often than males.

I've got butterflies in my stomach.

Flustered

These sayings could be used by almost anyone.

He's like a chook with its head cut off.

She has her knickers in a knot. (also for frustration)

Agitation/frustration

She has her knickers in a knot.

He had a tanti. (tantrum)

She had a hissy fit.

Annoyance or irritation

Almost anyone could say the following to any other person to describe someone else.

He's a pain in the neck.

The following sayings are quite vulgar and therefore would not be used by everyone and would not be used in polite company.

She's a pain in the arse.

It gives me the shits.

Disbelief

The first term below is used by older people and people from rural areas more than others. All terms mean that the speaker does not believe the other person.

Don't come the raw prawn with me. (Aus)

Don't give me that. (Aus)

My foot!

As if! (Aus)

Yeah right!

You've got to be joking.

Overconfidence

The following terms are commonly used to describe someone else. You might even tell the person, 'You've got tickets on yourself,' which in certain contexts could be very insulting.

She's got tickets on herself. (Aus)

She's cocky.

He's over the top.

He's up himself.

She's over the top (or OTT). (NZ)

Defiance

The following sayings are very defiant, and would not be used with people who you hold in high regard. One would usually use these terms when describing to a third party what it is that they do not want to do.

It will be a cold day in hell when I'll . . .

It will be over my dead body.

Hell will freeze over before I . . .

To no longer care

The following are very commonly used, especially by younger people.

I'm over it. (Aus)

I have moved on.

To forget about things (deliberately) (i.e. denial)

The following sayings could be used by anyone, but would be most likely used by older people.

It's all under the table.

Sweep it under the carpet.

Feeling alien and/or out of place

The following sayings are quite common.

I felt like a fish out of water.

She stuck out like a sore thumb.

The following saying is a very old-fashioned saying and therefore would be used more often by people from older generations.

I felt like a shag on a rock. (Aus)

Additional colloquialisms

Drug and alcohol-related terms

Smoking

The following terms could be used by almost anybody to describe their own or another's heavy smoking.

He smokes like a train.

She smokes like a chimney.

The term 'smoke-o' is often used to describe a break taken in the workday to smoke.

He's gone for a smoke-o.

Cigarettes

Common terms for cigarettes include 'cancer sticks', 'fags', 'ciggies', 'durries' (Aus), 'darts' (Aus) and 'poles' (NZ). These terms could be used by almost anyone, although 'fags' is more common. 'Durries' and 'darts' would be used mostly by rural youth (they are uncommon terms).

Drinking

The following saying could be used by anyone to describe someone who drinks a great deal of alcohol. It is usually used in relation to a third person, and not usually used to describe oneself.

She drinks like a fish.

A 'tinnie' means a can of beer and could be used by anyone. 'Amber fluid' means beer, and could be used by anyone, but is mostly used by older people. A 'shout' is a very common term, and means it is someone's turn to buy a drink for everyone in the group.

Pass me a tinnie.

I could do with an amber fluid.

It's OK—it's my shout.

Hotel

The terms 'waterhole' or 'pub' are usually used by older people. 'Bottle shop' (Aus) or 'Bottle-o' (Aus) refer to a shop that sells alcohol.

Affected by alcohol

Anyone might use the following terms, although not to everyone, as they are vulgar. Younger people use them more often than older people.

She's as pissed as a newt.

She's as pissed as a fart.

He is a pisshead.

He's had a skin full.

The following sayings are more polite, and are used more by older people.

She's as drunk as a skunk.

She's as full as a boot. (Aus)

He's off his face.

He's as full as a bull. (NZ)

She's as drunk as a lord.

She's plastered.

He's off his trolley.

To give up using drugs or alcohol

Common terms are to 'dry out', 'go cold turkey', 'on the wagon' and 'detox'. Anyone might use these terms to describe their own or someone else's experience. 'Drying out' usually refers to abstaining from drinking alcohol after having had considerable quantities over a long period of time. 'Going cold turkey' is usually used to describe the immediate cessation of any drug-taking after having used it for some time.

Affected by drugs in general

The sayings below are usually understood by all age groups, but are mostly used by younger people to describe their own or someone else's experience. Usually, these sayings would not be used to describe alcohol intoxication, although 'smashed', 'off my face' and 'out of it' might in some cases. They are usually used when talking about other drugs, both legal and illegal, including marijuana, heroin and prescription drugs taken with alcohol.

I was out of it.

I was whacked.

He was as high as a kite.

He was wasted.

She was smashed.

She was spun out.

I was off my face.

I was off the planet.

He was stoned.

He was bent.

She was off her head.

She was spaced out.

Additional colloquialisms

Body parts

Head

Terms used for the head include 'noggin', 'scone', 'nut' and 'swede' (NZ). The last two words are old-fashioned and would not ordinarily be used by younger people.

Heart

The terms 'ticker' and 'old ticker' are used by older people.

Breasts

The terms 'tits', 'boobs', 'titties' and 'boobies' could be used by anyone. The terms could be quite crude, depending on the context.

Penis

The terms 'old fella', 'cock', 'dick' and 'prick' could be used by anyone, although they are quite crude. The terms 'doodle', 'pee pee' (Aus) and 'willy' are most often used with children.

Testicles

The term 'balls' could be used by anyone. 'Nuts' and 'knackers' are quite crude.

Scrotum

The term 'scrote' could be used as an insult and is crude.

Specific injuries/conditions related to body parts

She has a gammy leg. (immobile or painful leg)

He has a dicky heart. (cardiovascular disease)

He has stuffed his knee. (injured his knee)

I've put my back out. (sore back)

I have a tummy ache. (stomach ache)

I've got a splitting head.

My head is pounding. (throbbing headache)

I have a frog in my throat. (sore throat that affects the voice)

My nose is blocked. (nasal congestion)

I'm stuffed up. (nasal/sinus congestion)

I have a crick in my neck. (sore neck)

I have problems with my water works. (incontinence or other problem with urinating)

I'm straining the spuds. (difficulty urinating (male))

I have front passage problems. (trouble with the urinary tract, usually passing urine)

I have the clap. (sexually transmitted disease)

I have trouble down there. (problem with the genitals)

I have sore private parts. (sore genitals)

I have a back passage problem. (trouble with the anus, usually with passing faeces)

I have sore boobs. (painful breasts)

She has something nasty. (cancer)

She has something sinister. (cancer)

He has the big C. (Aus) (cancer)

Is it the C-word? (cancer)

Additional colloquialisms

____

____

____

Body functions

Breathing

The following all refer to being short of breath (being breathless) and are used by most people.

I am out of puff.

I can't catch my breath.

I am out of breath.

I can't get my breath.

Faeces and defecation

Terms used for faeces include 'shit', 'poo', 'number twos', 'crap', 'to lay a cable' (Aus), and 'to push one out' (Aus). Poo is more polite, and is used especially with children.

The term 'turd' is often used by younger people and is quite vulgar.

In hospitals, it is common for health professionals to ask the following questions (both refer to defecation).

Have you used your bowels?

Have you been?

Diarrhoea

Most people experiencing diarrhoea would use one of these terms to the doctor if they did not say 'diarrhoea'.

I've got the runs.

I have the trots.

The following saying is vulgar, but it might be used with the doctor.

I have the shits.

Constipation

I haven't been.

I can't go.

I haven't used my bowels.

Urine and urination

Terms for urine/urination include 'piss', 'pee', 'wee', 'wee-wee', 'number ones', 'wizz', 'have a wee', 'pass water' and mimi (mostly Māori NZ). 'Have a wee', 'wee', 'wee-wee' and 'number one' are terms that might be used with children. 'Pass water' is usually used with older people.

Toileting

'Spend a penny' is most likely to be used by older people. 'Visit the bathroom' or 'go to the bathroom' are very commonly used.

I'm going to powder my nose.

I'm going to spend a penny.

I'm going to visit the bathroom.

I'm going to visit the little boys'/girls' room.

Where is the bathroom?

Where is the loo?

To look at something

The terms 'to look' and 'have a gander' are old-fashioned and used mostly by older people.

The terms 'check it out', 'have a perve' (crude), 'have/take a squiz' and 'have a sticky/a sticky beak' are used by almost everyone.

To sit down

The following colloquialisms are common and used by everyone, but especially by older people. A 'pew' is the name for the seats the congregation sits on in a church.

Take a load off your feet.

Pull up a pew.

Grab a seat.

To vomit

The following are all common colloquial terms for vomiting: 'throw up'; 'chuck up'; 'spew'; 'chunder'; 'chuck'; and 'puke'. The most polite one is probably 'throw up'. Younger people would use the other terms more often than older people.

The sayings 'technicolour yawn' and 'make a call on the big white telephone' are much less common. Usually, only younger people would use these, and probably not in a healthcare setting, but rather in conversation with each other.

Pregnancy

Many people would simply say that they were or another person was 'pregnant', but the following terms could also be used. They might be used by any age group and could be used with the healthcare professional.

She's got a bun in the oven.

She's up the spout.

She's up the duff.

He's knocked her up.

She's preggers.

She's with child.

Hapu. (mostly Māori NZ)

She's in the family way.

She's expecting.

She's due in a few weeks.

To fall asleep/be sleeping

The following are all quite polite terms and are very common colloquialisms for sleeping: 'out like a light'; 'dropped off'; 'dead to the world'; 'nodded off'; 'had forty winks'; and 'sound asleep'.

Overweight

Terms that mean overweight include 'tubby', 'fat as a pig', 'porky' and 'chubby'. The latter terms are ones that might be used to describe yourself or a third person, but would not be used to someone's face if talking about them, as they are quite insulting. 'Tubby' is not quite so rude.

Menstruation

Terms used for menstruation include 'period', 'monthlies', 'periods' and 'that time of the month'. Australian women do not usually say that they are 'menstruating'. Most often they will say they have their 'period' or 'periods' or that it is 'that time of the month'. These terms are considered to be quite polite and a person would very often say this to a health professional.

Sometimes, menstruation is referred to as the 'rags' or being 'on the rags'. This is considered to be very crude and would definitely not be used in polite circles. A patient may use this term with a health professional.

The following terms are less common, and very old-fashioned: 'the curse'; 'the red flag is flying' (Aus); 'the visitor'; and 'monthly visitor'.

Having many children

The colloquialism 'they breed like rabbits' is usually used in a derogatory sense, as rabbits in Australia are considered to be a pest. However, the term is quite common and would be used by a wide cross-section of people.

Flatulence

The terms 'passing wind','passing gas', 'breaking wind' and 'pop/pop off' are seen as fairly polite. 'Pop' and 'pop off' are often used with children. A patient would say this to the doctor.

The terms 'fart' and 'farting' are more vulgar, although they are very common and most people would use them. A patient may say this to the doctor.

Death

All of the following sayings for death are very common. More often out of respect for the dead person, a more polite term such as 'passed away' might be used, but not necessarily.

She's as dead as a doornail.

She's as stiff as a board.

He's kicked the bucket.

He's 6 foot under.

He carked it.

He snuffed it.

She's pushing up daisies.

He's gone.

Originating from wartime, the following saying means that the person put up a fight with their illness or injury before they died. This term is not so common.

He died with his boots on.

Sensations

Pain

My leg is sore.

My back is killing me.

It hurts like hell.

It is agony.

I can't stand it. (refers to severity of pain, not legs or standing/walking)

Numbness

Everybody uses the following term to describe the sensation of tingling and numbness, usually in the limbs. A patient would certainly say this to the doctor or other healthcare professional.

I have pins and needles.

Muscular tension

The following sayings could be used by almost anyone. The term 'stiff' is not usually used to refer to a single muscle; rather, it is used to describe a limb or region or whole body.

I'm as stiff as a board.

I have knots in my neck.

My neck is tight.

Hunger

I'm starving.

I could eat a horse.

I'm ravenous.

I'm famished.

Thirst

I'm as dry as a chip. (Aus)

I'm dying of thirst.

Additional colloquialisms

____

____

____

People and relationships

Husband

The following terms are common: 'the old man'; 'the other half'; 'the better half'; 'hubby'; and 'Dad'. Older people use these terms more often than younger people.

Wife

Terms used for 'wife' include 'the missus', 'the little woman', 'mother', 'the other half' and 'the better half'. Older people use these terms more often than younger people.

Relatives

Terms used for 'relatives' include the 'rellies', 'the family', 'rels' and 'rellos'. 'The in-laws' refers to parents-in-law, brothers-in-law and sisters-in-law.

Women

The terms 'chicks' and 'birds' are not as common as they once were, but some people still use these words in conversation. They are considered sexist.

'Sheila' (Aus) is a very old-fashioned Australian term (actually a female name) and older males still refer to women as 'sheilas'. You would hear people from rural areas say this more than people from the city. It is considered sexist.

The term 'Doris' (NZ) is a very old-fashioned term (actually a female name), used mostly by older males.

'Rough' people

The following are fairly common terms used by almost anyone to describe others perceived to be lower in social standing than oneself: 'yobbos'; 'riff-raff'; 'hoons'; 'ferals' (Aus); and 'bogans' (Aus). 'Yobbos' and 'hoons' usually refer to males only.

Additional colloquialisms

Health professionals

Psychiatrist

Lay people will often refer to a psychiatrist as 'a shrink'.

Doctor

The terms 'quack' and 'the Doc' are used most often by older people or those from rural areas.

Additional colloquialisms

Developmental stages

Children

The following are quite common terms for children and might be used by almost anyone: 'rug rats'; 'ankle biters'; 'sprogs'; 'kids'; 'tackers'; 'scone grabbers' (NZ) and 'nippers'.

Adolescence

Many parents and grandparents will talk about the teenage years as being a 'stage'.

> It's just a stage he's going through.
>
> She's at that awkward age.
>
> It's a teenage thing.

Older people

Older people might be referred to as 'oldies' or 'geris' (from geriatric).

Additional colloquialisms

Absence (due to illness or not)

To miss work

The following are very common ways of saying that you did not go to work, either because you were unwell or because you pretended to be unwell.

> I'm going to take a sickie.
>
> I'm taking a mental health day. (often to have a day off due to stress)

To miss school

'Wag', 'wagging' and 'bunk' are very common terms used by school children who do not attend school when they are not ill.

Additional colloquialisms

Miscellaneous

Difficult situation

The following sayings are very vulgar and would not be used in polite company.

He's up shit creek without a paddle.

I'm in the shit.

The following sayings are all quite polite and used by nearly everyone.

It's all downhill from here.

It's all going south from here. (Aus)

I'm in a spot of bother.

I'm in a bind.

To be reprimanded

The following sayings refer to being in trouble or being disciplined (as a consequence of behaviour).

She's on the mat. (NZ)

I've been hauled over the coals.

To be misled

The following are all reasonably common sayings used by a variety of people for different situations.

I've been led on a wild goose chase.

In the end, it was a red herring.

She's been given a bum steer.

To misunderstand

The following is a reasonably common expression.

She's got the wrong end of the stick.

To finish

The following are common sayings used by many people of different backgrounds in many different situations.

I'm home and hosed.

It's over and done with.

I'm signed off.

I'm done.

That's all done and dusted.

To leave

Many people would simply say that they 'left', but all the terms below are common. In describing a broken marriage, it is not uncommon to hear one partner say that the other 'shot through', 'ran off' or 'ran out'. The sayings are used by a wide cross-section of people in different situations.

He's going to shoot through.

He's going to vamoose.

She's going to do a disappearing act. (Aus)

He's gone AWOL. (absent without leave) (Aus)

He's going to run out.

She's going to run off.

Cheers, I'll run along now.

I'm heading off.

To tell someone to leave

Why don't you bugger off? (crude)

Piss off. (crude)

Nick off.

Make yourself scarce.

Get lost.

To complain

The terms to 'whinge' and to 'sook' mean to complain. Common terms include 'having a whinge', 'having a sook', 'to be a whinger' and 'to be a sook'.

To relax

The terms to 'wind down' (Aus), to 'let your hair down' and 'unwind' mean to relax.

To insist

To 'put your foot down' means to insist on something.

To like another person

The terms to 'hit it off' and to 'get on like a house on fire' mean to get along with.

They got along really well.

They hit it off.

They get on like a house on fire.

Working hard

The following colloquialisms would usually be used by older people and are common. To 'crack the whip' means that one person has strongly encouraged another to work hard.

I have my nose to the grindstone.

Pull your finger out.

He is going hell for leather.

Use some elbow grease.

I'm flat strapped.

I'm flat out.

I have my head down, bum up.

He cracked the whip.

I'm going flat out.

I'm going flat tack.

It's full on.

She's working like a slave.

Lazy

The terms 'bludger' (Aus) and 'slacker' (Aus) are used by many people. 'Slack arse' (Aus) is more vulgar. 'Bludger' is derogatory and indicates extreme laziness. 'Dole-bludger' indicates that a person is unemployed and survives on welfare payments.

Clothes

'Gear', 'outfit', 'clobber' (Aus) and 'kit' (Aus) all refer to clothes. Kit is used by older people.

Not wearing uniform

'Mufti', 'civvies' (Aus) and 'free dress' mean no uniform or casual clothing.

Underwear

The following refer to underpants: 'underdaks' (male); 'jocks' (male); 'panties' (female); 'undies' (both genders); 'knickers' (females or both genders for children); and 'boxers' (boxer shorts) (male).

'Smalls' refers to underwear (including bras) and is often used by older people.

Rural areas

The following terms refer to rural areas: 'out in the sticks' (Aus); 'in the bush' (Aus); 'woop woop'; 'out in the middle of nowhere' (Aus); 'in Timbuktu' (Aus); 'back of beyond' (Aus); and 'back of Burke' (an outback town) (Aus).

Cities or metropolitan areas

Cities are often referred to as 'the big smoke'.

Food

'Macca's' is often used by younger people for McDonald's. Other terms for food include 'brekkie' (breakfast), 'brunch' (a combined late breakfast/early lunch), 'tea' (dinner or the evening meal), 'junk food' (unhealthy food), 'tucker' (food) and a 'feed' (a meal).

Bad smell

The words 'pong', 'stink', 'wiffy' and 'stench' are often used for a bad smell.

Additional colloquialisms

____

____

____

Phrasal verbs

By M Bernadette Hally

Phrasal verbs are used very frequently in English. Some phrasal verbs are used in healthcare (e.g. put up the IV fluid) or refer specifically to health (e.g. come down with a cold), while others are used in general conversation and can be applied to healthcare (e.g. take off your jewellery before surgery). In Table 8.1, where a health-related phrasal verb also has a common usage meaning, both forms are given. Some of these phrasal verbs are also listed in the colloquialisms section of this chapter above.

Additional phrasal verbs

____

____

____

TABLE 8.1 Phrasal verbs

Phrasal verb	Meaning	Example
Bring on	To cause, start or induce	The patient thought that eating spicy food had brought on his indigestion. This drug will bring on labour (as in birth).
Bring up (1) See: Throw up	To vomit	He brought up his dinner.
Bring up (2)	Common usage: to raise, mention (in conversation)	He did not bring up his history of depression.
Come down with See: Go down with, Pick up	To contract, develop	He came down with pneumonia.
Come round/come around	To regain consciousness	He came round after half an hour.

(Continued)

TABLE 8.1 Phrasal verbs—*cont'd*

Phrasal verb	Meaning	Example
Come through See: Get through; Make it, Pull through	To survive, manage	She came through after the operation.
Come to	Common usage: to awaken	I came to when the alarm rang.
Cut down	To reduce	The doctor advised him to cut down his fat intake.
Cut out	To stop, cease, avoid	She must cut out gluten in her diet.
Dose up	To medicate, take medication or preparations (for health)	He was dosed up with analgesia after surgery. At the first sign of a cold, she doses up on Vitamin C.
Draw back	To aspirate (with a syringe) (this is the action when the plunger is removed from the barrel)	To deflate the balloon in the indwelling catheter, the nurse connected a syringe to the port and drew back the water.
Draw up	To fill the syringe with a drug (from a container)	The clinical teacher watched the student draw up the antibiotic from the glass vial.
Drop off See: Nod off	To fall asleep	I dropped off at 10 o'clock.
Fill in	To write or document	He filled in the fluid balance chart.
Fill out	To write or document	She filled out the incident report.
Fill up	To fill or refill	The wound drainage bag filled up quickly.
Get hold of	To contact	The nurse will get hold of the surgeon and tell him that the patient's wound is haemorrhaging.
Get over (1)	To recover	He will get over the flu.
Get over (2)	Common usage: to stop caring/worrying	Get over it!
Get through See: Come through, Make it through, Pull through	To survive or recover	She got through the operation.
Give up	To stop, cease	He has given up smoking.
Go down with See: Come down with, Pick up	To contract, develop	I don't want to go down with gastro.
Go through (1)	To experience (usually refers to a negative or difficult situation)	He has gone through a lot since his wife died. The patient does not want to go through that again.

TABLE 8.1 Phrasal verbs—*cont'd*

Phrasal verb	Meaning	Example
Go through (2) See: Run out (1), Run through (2)	To finish, be completed	The IV has gone through on time.
Hand over	To communicate information (for continued action)	The nurse in the recovery room will hand over the patient before he returns to the ward.
Make it through See: Come through, Get through, Pull through	To survive, manage	He made it through the chemotherapy without any nausea.
Out of . . .(1)	To be without, lacking, insufficient	I am out of breath (breathless). I am out of puff (breathless). I am out of condition (unwell, unfit).
Out of it (1)	To be unconscious, or confused (often as a result of drug or alcohol use)	He was out of it after he had narcotic analgesia. She was recently diagnosed with dementia, but her son said she has been out of it for many years.
Out of . . ./Out of it (2)	Common usage: to no longer be performing an activity or practice	She was a nurse, but she has been out of it for 10 years. The lecturer had been out of the clinical setting for 2 years.
Pass out	To lose consciousness (also to faint)	The student passed out while observing the lumbar puncture.
Pick up (1) See: Come down with, Go down with	To contract, develop	She picked up a cold.
Pick up (2)	To improve	He picked up after he started eating and drinking.
Pull out	To remove (from an internal site)	He pulled out the intravenous cannula.
Pull through See: Come through, Get through, Make it through	To survive	She pulled through after the accident.
Put in (1)	To insert	The nurse put in the indwelling catheter.
Put in (2)	To give, apply oneself or to try	She put in many hours this week. He has put in with his study this semester.
Put on (1)	To apply (can also mean to wear)	I will put a bandage on your ankle. Put on this gown before surgery.
Put on (2)	To pretend, deceive or exaggerate—often related to illness, disability or pain	She is putting on that limp. I saw her walking normally a minute ago!

(Continued)

TABLE 8.1 Phrasal verbs—*cont'd*

Phrasal verb	Meaning	Example
Put on (3)	To gain (amount)	She has put on 6 kg since admission.
Put up (1)	To raise	The student nurse put up the IV flask. Put your feet up to reduce the oedema.
Put up (2)	To tolerate	I don't know how she puts up with the pain.
Run down	To be exhausted, lacking energy and at risk of becoming unwell	She was very run down before she became sick.
Run out (1) See: Go through (2), Run through (2)	To finish, be completed	The IV has run out. We have run out of drug orders.
Run out (2) See: Take off (2)	Common usage: to leave (responsibilities, a person or a relationship)	He ran out on his wife and children.
Run through (1)	To explain.	The clinical teacher ran through the procedure with the student nurse.
Run through (2) See: Go through (2), Run out (1)	To finish, be completed	The IV has run through too quickly.
Sew up	To suture	That wound will need to be sewn up.
Take down	To remove (a dressing)	Let's take down the dressing and assess the suture line.
Take off (1)	To remove	Take off your jewellery before having an X-ray. The doctor will take off that lesion.
Take off (2) See: Run out (2)	Common usage: to leave (often refers to responsibilities, a person or a relationship)	She took off with another man.
Take off (3)	Common usage: to depart	He took off at lunchtime.
Take out	To remove	I will take out his intercostal catheters.
Take up	To start (a practice or habit)	She has taken up eating breakfast.
Throw up See: Bring up (1)	To vomit	He threw up after lunch.
Top up	To add more	I have topped up the enteral feed.
Wear out	To age, need replacement	The doctor says my hip joint has worn out.

CHAPTER HIGHLIGHTS

- Informal language is used in everyday communication.
- You will need to be familiar with the health-related informal terms and expressions used by patients and staff in healthcare settings.
- You will need to ask the meanings of any expressions you do not understand.

- Becoming familiar with the colloquialisms related to healthcare will be useful for your nursing practice.
- Understanding and using common phrasal verbs in the healthcare setting will improve your communication.

Self-test questions

1. Listen to the CD Part 1—Audio, 'Pronunciation of colloquialisms' (A1) and 'Pronunciation of phrasal verbs' (A2).
2. Note any new colloquialisms or phrasal verbs you hear (in conversations with local people, during clinical placement or at your workplace, on radio or television) or read, in the relevant spaces in this chapter.
3. Update your 'Language list' (R2) on the CD Part 3—Reader resources.

References

Chur-Hansen A 2005 Talking about health and illness: Australian colloquialisms and informal English. Unpublished class notes. Department of Psychiatry, University of Adelaide, Adelaide, South Australia

Chur-Hansen A, Elliott T, Supple L 2006 Talking about health and illness: Australian slang. Unpublished class notes. Adaptation of Chur-Hansen A 2005 Talking about health and illness: Australian colloquialisms and informal English, Adelaide to Outback. Department of Psychiatry, University of Adelaide, Adelaide, South Australia

CHAPTER 9

Healthcare jargon

'It is hard to remember all the terminology . . . it takes much practice!'

Femida, Uganda

CHAPTER OUTLINE

LEARNING OBJECTIVES

1. Become familiar with the jargon used in healthcare in Australia or New Zealand.
2. Develop an understanding of the medical terminology used in healthcare in Australia or New Zealand through focused self-directed learning.
3. Develop an understanding of the abbreviations used in healthcare in Australia or New Zealand through focused self-directed learning.
4. Recognise the limitations to the use of abbreviations.
5. Become familiar with the acronyms used in healthcare in Australia or New Zealand.

Key terms (are in bold in the text)

abbreviations
acronyms
colloquialisms
jargon
terminology

In Australia and New Zealand, health professionals use **jargon** extensively. You will need to be familiar with medical and nursing jargon to communicate with your colleagues, and to be able to care for your patients. Unlike some **colloquialisms**, you will be expected to use all parts of jargon—medical terminology, abbreviations and acronyms—appropriately in your nursing practice.

This chapter will provide you with resources for self-directed learning and recommend strategies for developing your competence in the use of jargon.

When you hear or read unfamiliar jargon, remember to ask the person who has said it, what the term means. (See Ch 2 for hints on developing your English and 'nursing English'.) You could say: 'I am not familiar with that term. Could you please repeat it?' or 'What does that term mean?' If the person cannot explain the meaning to you, ask a teacher or colleague or use a dictionary or other language resource (such as a list of acceptable abbreviations at the clinical facility). You should write the new expression and its meaning in your 'Language list' (R2) on the CD Part 3—Reader resources.

Terminology

There are a number of resources that address the topic of medical **terminology**. It is strongly recommended that you consult the Australian/New Zealand medical terminology text listed in the 'Recommended reading' (Nicol & Walker 2007) and that you complete the 'Medical terminology self-directed learning package' (R10) on the CD Part 3—Reader resources. Remember also that developing your English language skills, particularly your academic and professional 'nursing' English (as recommended in Ch 2), will assist you to understand and use medical terminology competently.

Abbreviations

Abbreviations are sometimes truncated—shortened—forms of words, or the initials of words. If the initials form a new pronounceable word or the letters of the initials are pronounced (when speaking), these abbreviations are called **acronyms**. Table 9.1 highlights the differences between abbreviations and acronyms.

It is important to be familiar with standard abbreviations, as you will frequently need to understand and use these. Throughout this text, common standard abbreviations are provided (in brackets after the full term).

While the use of abbreviations is a common practice, it is effective only if the meaning of the abbreviation is interpreted correctly. Using your own abbreviations could be dangerous, if the meaning of 'your' abbreviation was not interpreted correctly. It is important to *use only standard abbreviations and those approved for use in the clinical facility*. Most clinical facilities have a list of acceptable abbreviations and sometimes these are adapted for use in individual wards/units/areas.

Comprehensive lists of abbreviations and their meanings are provided in the Australian/New Zealand medical terminology text listed in the 'Recommended reading' (Nicol & Walker 2007). This excellent resource has the abbreviations listed by topic in each chapter. It is strongly recommended that you complete the 'Healthcare abbreviations self-directed learning package' (R11) on the CD Part 3—Reader resources.

TABLE 9.1 Comparing abbreviations and acronyms

Element of jargon	Definition	Types	Examples		
			Written form	*Pronunciation*	*Meaning*
Abbreviation	Shortened form of a word or words	Truncated (shortened) form of a word	abdo	'abdo'	Abdomen, abdominal
			gynae	'gynae'	Gynaecology, gynaecological
		Initials of words, which are used only in writing and are *not* used in speech	OA	*Not* used in speech	Osteoarthritis
			ATSP	*Not* used in speech	Asked to see patient
Acronyms	A type of abbreviation	True acronyms: initials of words that form a *new pronounceable word*	NIDDM	'niddm'	Non-insulin dependent diabetes mellitus
			CAT (scan)	'cat'	Computerised axial tomography (scan)
		Other acronyms: initials of words where the *initials are pronounced*	ECG	'E-C-G'	Electrocardiogram, electrocardiograph
			RN	'R-N'	Registered nurse

Acronyms

Acronyms are commonly used in nursing, and you need to be able to use them confidently. In addition to knowing its meaning, you must be able to pronounce the acronym correctly. Remember that true acronyms form a new pronounceable word (e.g. NIDDM), while others are pronounced by saying the name of the initials (e.g. ECG). A list of acronyms is provided on the CD. See the CD Part 2—Transcripts, 'Pronunciation of acronyms' (T3). To hear how to pronounce the acronyms, listen to the CD Part 1—Audio, 'Pronunciation of acronyms' (A3).

CHAPTER HIGHLIGHTS

- Jargon is used extensively among health professionals.
- You will need to be competent in the use of jargon—medical terminology, abbreviations and acronyms.
- To develop your competence in using medical terminology, improve your English language and complete focused learning activities.
- To avoid errors and confusion with abbreviations, use only standard abbreviations or those approved by the clinical facility.
- To develop your competence in using abbreviations, complete focused learning activities.

- To develop your competence in using and pronouncing acronyms, complete focused learning activities.

Self-test questions

1. Why is it important for international nurses and students to be competent in the use of jargon?
2. Discuss the important considerations for using abbreviations.
3. Listen to the CD Part 1—Audio, 'Pronunciation of acronyms' (A3).
4. Complete the 'Medical terminology self-directed learning package' (R10) on the CD Part 3—Reader resources.
5. Complete the 'Healthcare abbreviations self-directed learning package' (R11) on the CD Part 3—Reader resources.
6. Update your 'Language list' with any new jargon (medical terminology, abbreviations and acronyms) you hear or read using your 'Language list' (R2) on the CD Part 3—Reader resources.

Recommended reading

Nicol J, Walker S (eds) 2007 The language of medicine. Elsevier Australia, Sydney. This citation is for the Australian and New Zealand edition adapted from: Chabner D 2004 The language of medicine. Elsevier St Louis. The text cover of the cited text reads as follows: The language of medicine: Australian and New Zealand edition by Davi-Ellen Chabner. The editors are not noted at all on the cover of the text, so it will *appear different* if you are looking for a copy of the book. The citation details are on the inside front cover of the cited text.

PART 4

Communicating in nursing

CHAPTER 10

Verbal communication

'I am very scared about handovers when I am working in a hospital. It seems so fast! I know I must make sure my English is very good, and practise listening and speaking as much as possible because I want to be a safe nurse.'

Gigi, Thailand

CHAPTER OUTLINE

LEARNING OBJECTIVES

1. Discuss the purposes of verbal communication.
2. Discuss the principles of verbal communication.
3. Describe the key aspects of communication.
4. Describe the situations where nurses use verbal communication in nursing practice.
5. Describe the types, purposes and format of verbal handovers in nursing practice.
6. Define therapeutic relationships and therapeutic communication.
7. Outline the key skills required for therapeutic communication.

Key terms (are in bold in the text)

communication
confidentiality
non-verbal communication
privacy

cultural sensitivity
endorsement
handover
therapeutic communication
therapeutic relationships
verbal communication

Verbal communication can be a difficult skill for international nurses and nursing students, as it requires proficiency in the various 'types' of English used in clinical settings. This includes general formal and informal English language skills, as well as academic English and formal and informal professional 'nursing' English language skills (which are discussed in detail in Ch 2). In nursing practice, verbal communication skills are used in an extensive range of situations, with a variety of people. This chapter focuses on the key verbal interactions used in the clinical setting, and provides a brief overview of therapeutic communication.

Verbal communication

It is a nursing competency requirement that you can communicate effectively in English. To be a safe and competent nurse and nursing student, you *must* be able to demonstrate excellent **verbal communication** skills. (See Ch 5 for a detailed discussion of nursing competency standards.)

Purpose of verbal communication

Communication is the process where messages are conveyed from person to person. Verbal communication involves the use of the spoken word, and is often accompanied by non-verbal communication (or body language).

Communication is an essential skill in nursing. Verbal communication facilitates the development of relationships—with patients and colleagues—and allows for sharing of information about patient care (Stein-Parbury 2009 Ch 23). Poor communication or failure to communicate can have serious consequences in nursing.

Principles of verbal communication

While there is greater emphasis on the legal requirements of documentation than there is on verbal communication, certain principles are equally relevant in verbal communication (see Table 10.1).

Cultural sensitivity is important in verbal interactions, as language and culture are strongly related (Antai-Otong 2006, Dowd et al 2009 Ch 8, Walton & Marriott 2008 pp 29–30). It is important to understand the implications of language in healthcare for Indigenous people. The New South Wales (NSW) state health department has prepared a document for health professionals to assist them in using appropriate language when communicating with Indigenous Australians. It is recommended that you obtain a copy of this publication, listed in the 'Recommended reading' (New South Wales Health 2004). Chapter 6 addresses issues related to Māori health, and provides examples of culturally appropriate care and examples of Māori terminology.

It is also essential that nurses protect patients' **privacy** and **confidentiality** in all verbal communication.

TABLE 10.1 Principles of verbal communication

Principles	Explanation/rationale
Accurate	Be specific and correct.
Factual	Be truthful.
Objective	Avoid subjective comments or personal opinions that reflect negatively on other people (patients or colleagues). Avoid labelling, stereotypes and derogatory terms to describe others.
Complete	Do not avoid verbal communication. Avoid omissions (do not leave out important information). If care is omitted, state why.
Concise	Be brief. Avoid repetition and do not routinely report normal data or information recorded on standard documents. Repeat only unusual or significant data in handover.
Contemporaneous (timely)	Report deterioration in the patient's condition, clinical emergencies, abnormal findings or errors immediately.
Privacy and confidentiality	Nurses must ensure that all verbal communication about patients remains private and confidential, according to the laws governing privacy and confidentiality of health information. Communicate information only to relevant and appropriate health professionals (involved in the patient's care). Ensure that conversations about patients are conducted in private and cannot be overheard.
Document key verbal communication	All verbal reports (e.g. advising a doctor that the patient has chest pain) and referrals (e.g. to a social worker) should be documented.
Culturally sensitive	Care should be taken to ensure that verbal interactions are culturally sensitive.

Forms of communication

Non-verbal communication is often used in conjunction with verbal communication. The key aspects of both forms of communication are outlined in Table 10.2, along with the nursing implications and examples.

?| QUESTION FOR REFLECTION

Are any key aspects of communication different in your culture?

Verbal communication in nursing practice

All verbal communication in nursing practice should be courteous and polite. It should convey care and respect for the patient, and be accompanied by appropriate non-verbal communication.

Nurses communicate with patients/clients and their families/significant others (e.g. during admission interview, in therapeutic communication), with other nurses about patient care (e.g. during **handover**, also called **endorsement** in some countries) or

TABLE 10.2 Key aspects of communication

Key aspect	Comment	Examples
Verbal communication		
Vocabulary	Avoid the use of medical terminology and jargon with patients. Consider the patient's developmental stage and use appropriate vocabulary. Consider the patient's language background and use interpreters when needed.	You have a high temperature. *Not*: You are febrile.
Meaning (of vocabulary)	Shared meaning is essential for understanding. Certain words or terms could be interpreted as having a different meaning by the patient. Use common language and verify that the patient has understood what has been said.	Do you take any medications? *Not*: Do you take drugs?
Pace	Use a pace that is neither too slow nor too rapid.	
Tone	Intonation often reflects emotion and can alter the meaning of the message. Use an appropriate tone and aim to 'sound professional'.	
Clarity	Speak slowly. Enunciate clearly (say words distinctly). Use examples. Be concise.	Tell me about the pain. *Not*: Could you please give me a description of the onset, location and nature of the pain.
Timing	Ensure the patient is 'ready' for the message (note that pain and anxiety can prevent effective communication). In an emergency, ensure the communication is very clear and concise.	During an episode of acute chest pain: This tablet goes under the tongue and should help relieve the pain. *Not*: If you experience chest pain at home, sit down, place a tablet under the tongue, wait 5 minutes and, if the pain is not alleviated, take another tablet. If the pain has not gone after 15 minutes and a total of three tablets, call an ambulance.
Relevance	Ensure the message matches the patient's needs.	Your blood pressure is within the normal range.

TABLE 10.2 Key aspects of communication—*cont'd*

Key aspect	Comment	Examples
Relevance—*cont'd*		*Not*: Your blood pressure is within the normal range, but if it was too high you could be at risk of a stroke and a stroke could cause permanent disability or death.
Non-verbal communication		
Personal appearance	How one presents reflects personality, attitude, emotions, self-concept and health status. Aim to present yourself as a professional nurse.	Facilities often have a uniform policy to promote a professional image and ensure safety (e.g. occupational health and safety, infection control).
Posture and gait (walking style)		A patient who is walking very slowly could be experiencing pain.
Facial expression	The face is often very expressive. Smiling is universally understood to be positive. Grimacing indicates disgust or displeasure.	While changing the patient's colostomy bag, the nurse grimaces. (This is not appropriate non-verbal communication.) The nurse raises his eyebrows and rolls his eyes during the handover from another nurse. (This is not appropriate non-verbal communication and could be interpreted as boredom, disbelief, or general disrespect for his colleague.)
Eye contact	In Western culture, eye contact indicates readiness to communicate, engagement, attention, honesty and confidence. When people are positioned at the same eye level (or height), it promotes a sense of equality.	During an interview, the nurse rarely makes eye contact with the patient. The patient feels that the nurse is disinterested in her. The patient feels uncomfortable when the nurse is standing beside his chair, looking down at him. He feels more comfortable when he sits in the chair beside him and his eyes are at the same level as his.
Gestures	Use of the hands or facial features conveys a message. Guarding (protecting a part of the body with one's hands) often indicates pain. In Western culture, nodding the head indicates an affirmative response (i.e. yes) or agreement. Shaking the head (from side to side) indicates a negative response (i.e. no) or disagreement.	The patient points to his left knee to indicate the site of his pain.

(Continued)

TABLE 10.2 Key aspects of communication—*cont'd*

Key aspect	Comment	Examples
Sounds	Sounds generally indicate positive or negative emotion. Groaning or moaning can often be an indication of pain.	In the palliative care unit, the nurse notes that when placed in the left lateral position, the semi-conscious patient begins to moan.
Personal space and touch	Nursing care requires nurses to enter the patient's personal space and to touch parts of the patient's body. Great sensitivity is required and verbal consent should be obtained before touching certain parts of the body (e.g. genitals).	The student nurse is tentative when assisting the patient to have a shower, as she is unaccustomed to being in the personal space of a stranger.

Source: Adapted from Stein-Parbury 2005a pp 423–5.

professional issues (e.g. discussing a new procedure), with other health professionals (e.g. during a multidisciplinary team meeting or when referring the patient for review by another health professional) and with other (non-professional) staff in the healthcare setting (e.g. kitchen staff, when ordering a patient's meal).

In Australia and New Zealand, colleagues often refer to and address each other on a 'first name basis' (this means using given names). Many patients will also invite you to call them by their first names. It is not considered impolite to ask patients their preferred name, and this is usually done (and documented) as part of the admission interview.

Table 10.3 provides examples of appropriate verbal communication for a variety of situations in nursing practice. Listen to the CD to hear examples of verbal communication in clinical conversations (CD Part 1—Audio, 'Nursing conversations' (A4–A14) and 'Nursing handovers' (A15–A16)) and complete the activities and self-test questions in Part 7 to improve your verbal communication skills.

QUESTION FOR REFLECTION

Which aspects of nursing handover do you find most challenging and how can you develop your skills in this area?

Therapeutic communication

A **therapeutic relationship** is a unique healing relationship between health professional and person, where the goal is to promote the person's health, wellbeing and self-actualisation (Arnold 2007 p 200). **Therapeutic communication** is 'a specialized form of communication used in health settings to support, educate and empower people' (Arnold 2007 p 200) to meet health-related goals. Table 10.5 provides an overview of therapeutic communication skills. Further reading, study and supervised practice are recommended to develop skills in therapeutic communication. It is highly recommended that you read more about therapeutic communication from the source listed in the 'Recommended reading' (Stein-Parbury 2009).

? QUESTION FOR REFLECTION

Reflect on a situation—in a clinical setting if possible—when you felt that someone 'cared for' you. List the therapeutic communication skills that the other person demonstrated.

TABLE 10.3 Nursing conversations and handovers

Situation	Comment	Examples
Communicating with patients		
Introductions	When meeting the patient for the first time, or at the start of the shift, always introduce yourself. Address the patient by their preferred name (ask if unsure).	Good morning Mr Ho, my name is Kim. I am a third-year nursing student and I am working with Mary Benz and we will be looking after you today. Hello Grace, I'm Jocelyn and I am your nurse for this shift. Hello Frank, I'm Sam. I'm going to care for you again today.
Social conversation	You must be able to have a social conversation with your patient. Be informed about news and current affairs, be able to ask general questions about the patient, and be prepared to share some appropriate information about yourself. Avoid potentially sensitive topics (i.e. politics, religion or personal or intimate subjects, such as reason for marital status).	I see you are watching the basketball. In my country this is a popular sport. What is the weather forecast for tomorrow? You are a retired teacher. What did you teach? Was the baby I saw visiting you a grandchild? How old is she? These are beautiful flowers. What is the name of this flower in English? Is the book you are reading interesting?
Admission interview (see Box 10.1)	Be familiar with the documentation required for the nursing admission. Be able to formulate appropriate questions to obtain information. Explain that you are conducting an admission interview. Ensure that the patient consents for any other person (such as a spouse) to remain present before asking questions. Sometimes admission data is collected from other relevant people. You will need to arrange for any people to leave the room if it is not appropriate for them to be present.	I need to ask you some questions about your health history and check your temperature, pulse and blood pressure. Are you happy for me to do that now? I have come to ask you some questions about your medical history. I will also check your temperature, pulse and blood pressure. Are you happy for your son to remain here while I ask you about your health. Would you like your daughter to stay during the admission interview? Would you like her to help you answer any questions if you are unsure? I will be back in 10 minutes to ask you some questions. It will take about 15 minutes, and [to the visitor] I'll ask you to wait in the waiting room or perhaps I could direct you to the cafe.

(Continued)

TABLE 10.3 Nursing conversations and handovers—*cont'd*

Situation	Comment	Examples
Performing clinical skills	Explain the procedure clearly (especially if it is the first time the patient has had the procedure) and obtain the patient's (implied or express) consent.	I am going to take your blood pressure. Could you straighten your left arm and I will put the cuff around your arm. You will feel pressure on your arm as I pump up the cuff. Your blood pressure is 120 over 70. That's within the normal range.
Mobilising and positioning patients (see Box 10.2)	You will need to know the medical terminology or jargon (to read, document and communicate with your colleagues), as well as general formal and informal expressions for instructing patients.	I will help you turn over and lie on your left side. After your shower, we will sit you in the chair so you can have your breakfast. Could you look straight ahead while I check your pupils (eyes) with the torch? Turn your head to the left side, as far as you can.
Patient education	Ensure the patient is ready to learn. Use visual aids as appropriate. Be prepared to demonstrate skills. Check understanding by asking questions, and observing return demonstration.	I am going to show you how to change your colostomy bag. I will do it with you this time, and next time you can do it while I watch. [Demonstrate the procedure.] Here is the equipment you will need. Remove the old bag and place it in the rubbish bag. Clean the stoma. Place the new bag over the stoma. Make sure it is lined up properly. Do you have any questions?
Discharge	Often you will inform the patient of their planned discharge, and also provide discharge education.	Mrs Alonzo, you will be going home tomorrow. Discharge time is 10 a.m. Is someone able to collect you? [Yes, my daughter can.] Would you like me to call your daughter and tell her? [Yes, please.] We will give you some information before you go, including your follow-up appointment. Later tonight I will talk to you about caring for your wound. We have a discharge information sheet for you, so all this information will be written there too. We will also organise your medications and the pharmacist will explain these to you before you go.
Concluding conversation	When you leave the patient, it is appropriate to make a concluding remark. It is polite to say goodbye at the end of the shift.	I am going to check my other patients, but will be back in about half an hour. If you need anything, just use the call bell. It's here next to you. I am going to lunch. Park will look after you while I am gone. If you need anything, use the call bell. Good night Ms Venutti. I am going home now. I will see you in the morning. Carly will be your nurse tonight.

TABLE 10.3 Nursing conversations and handovers—*cont'd*

Situation	Comment	Examples
Telephone conversations	Always speak clearly, slowly and loudly enough to be heard on the telephone. State your name, the location (ward or facility) and your designation when answering or making calls. Write messages for staff and patients, including the names of callers and return numbers (as patients will not always have ready access to telephone directories). Be prepared to protect patient privacy and confidentiality (always be aware of the facility policy). In some cases, you should not even confirm whether the patient is present.	[Answering the telephone] Good morning, ward 7, this is Sheree de Souza, student nurse speaking. [Making calls] Hello, my name is Helen So. I am a registered nurse calling from Pleasant View Nursing Home. Caller: Can you tell me how Mr Jones is? Nurse: Could I ask who is calling please? Caller: It's Bill McKenzie. I am his cousin. Nurse: I am sorry. I cannot discuss patient information over the phone. I can take a message for you. Caller: Is Susie Lew in your ward? Nurse: Could I ask who is calling please? Caller: It's a friend. Nurse: I am sorry I cannot disclose any information over the phone. I will transfer you to patient enquiries.
Communicating with colleagues		
Telephone orders	Some medical orders, including medication orders are received by telephone and must always be documented. Check the facility policy regarding telephone orders for medications. Two registered nurses should listen to the order, write the order and sign the order (in the drug chart), and mention of a telephone order should be noted (in the progress notes).	RN James: Mrs Liu has chest pain. Could you give us a phone order please? Dr Huang: Mrs Liu can have 600 micrograms of anginine sublingually now. RN James: Thanks. You said that Mrs Liu can have 600 micrograms of anginine sublingually now. Dr Huang: That's correct. I'll get another RN to listen to that order as well. RN Han: It's Susan Han. Could you repeat the phone order please? Dr Huang: Mrs Liu can have 600 micrograms of anginine sublingually now. RN Han: Thank you. That was: Mrs Liu can have 600 micrograms of anginine sublingually now. We'll give her that now. Dr Huang: That's right. I'll be there to review her in about 15 minutes. Page me if the pain is not alleviated by the anginine. RN Han: Thanks, and we'll get you to sign the order when you get here. Dr Huang: Sure.
Reporting information	This is most often done in person or by telephone (and should also be documented). Nursing handover is a form of verbal reporting.	I paged you to tell you that Mrs Brown has not passed urine since 3 a.m. Mr Ng's wife has asked to see you. She is visiting him now. John Duncan's Hb is 102.

(Continued)

TABLE 10.3 Nursing conversations and handovers—*cont'd*

Situation	Comment	Examples
Referrals	Referrals to other health professionals are often made verbally (as well as being documented).	[To the speech pathologist] Could you see Mrs Jackson please? She seems to be having trouble swallowing and is choking on sips of water. [To the podiatrist] Would you please see Mr Lagaia? He has type 2 diabetes. [To the occupational therapist] Mrs Ng will need a domestic ADL assessment before we arrange her discharge.
Nursing handover (see Box 10.3)	Nursing handover is used extensively. Its purpose is to share patient information, staff debriefing and education. You will need to know medical terminology, abbreviations and jargon, as well as general formal and informal expressions, to understand and give verbal handovers.	See Table 10.4.

Box 10.1 Skills for conducting nursing admission interviews

During the nursing admission, the nurse conducts an interview with the patient, performs relevant physical assessments (e.g. cardiac assessment) and collects baseline assessment data (e.g. vital signs, weight and urinalysis). The nurse also reads the patient's file or medical record from previous admissions, an emergency service admission form (from the ambulance officers who transported the patient to hospital) or a referral letter from another health professional, if these documents are available.

Nursing admission interview forms could be organised in various ways. Some are organised according to body systems (e.g. respiratory, musculoskeletal, gastrointestinal), while others use a nursing assessment framework such as Gordon's functional health patterns (Gordon 2006). All nursing admission forms have sections for documenting demographic data, past medical history, allergies, information on the admission diagnosis, current problems, current medications and baseline assessment data.

Most facilities use standard questionnaire style forms for the nursing admission interviews (also known as the health history or admission assessment). These will list the type of information required, but do not list every question that you need to ask. For example, the chart might say 'Age', but you cannot simply say this to the patient! You will need to ask 'What is your date of birth?' or 'How old are you?' Listen to the CD Part 1—Audio, 'Nursing conversations—Admission interview' (A6). Complete the 'Nursing conversations' activities and self-test questions in Part 7, and complete the 'Admission interview self-directed learning package' (R8) on the CD Part 3—Reader resources.

Box 10.2 Skills for communicating about mobilising and positioning patients

Patient mobility and positioning is communicated between health professionals and documented using medical terminology, abbreviations and jargon. However, these terms are not always appropriate for using when assisting patients or instructing them about how to mobilise or position themselves. Typically, you will need to be able to use general and informal English to assist mobilising and positioning patients.

For example, the progress notes might state 'patient RIB supine'. You will need to understand that this means the patient is in bed, lying flat on his back. If a colleague asks you to help her move the patient into the right lateral position, you will need to understand that this means he will be repositioned to lie on his right side. If you are asking the patient to move from a supine to right lateral position, you will need to be able to tell him 'we are going to help you turn onto your right side'. Listen to the CD Part 1—Audio, 'Nursing conversations—Mobilising and positioning a patient' (A8). Complete the 'Nursing conversations' activities and the self-test questions in Part 7, and complete the 'Mobilising and positioning patients self-directed learning package' (R9) on the CD Part 3—Reader resources.

Box 10.3 Skills for nursing handover

Verbal handover is used extensively in nursing. Handovers (called endorsements in some countries) take place in a number of ways and occur when the nursing staff from the previous shift hand over to the staff on the next shift. Often this occurs in an office, and all oncoming staff listen to the handover about all the patients in the ward or unit. Sometimes, the nurse who has cared for the patient hands over only to the nurse allocated to care for the patient on the next shift. This often occurs at the bedside. Taped handovers are used in some facilities, and nurses record their handover during the shift, and the incoming staff listen to the tape at the start of their shift.

Apart from communicating key information about patients (see Table 10.4), nursing handover also provides an opportunity for staff debriefing and education (Chan 2001, Levett-Jones & Bourgeois 2007 p 155). Handover can be difficult for students and graduate nurses, as it requires a sound understanding of medical terminology, jargon and abbreviations, along with excellent English language skills. Developing your English language skills, listening to as many handovers as possible, and practising giving handovers, will improve your confidence in both listening to and delivering nursing handovers. Listen to the CD Part 1—Audio, 'Nursing handovers' (A15–A16). Complete the 'Nursing handovers' activities and the self-test questions in Part 7.

TABLE 10.4 Sample verbal handover format

Key information	Sample (as spoken)
Patient name/bed number	Mrs Summers/Bed 7
Age	78 years old
Medical diagnosis	With CCF
Day (of stay)	Admitted yesterday
Mobility	RIB with bathroom privileges
Assistance required	Assist with all ADLs
Other nursing diagnoses (problems) and care	SOB: requires continuous oxygen 2 litres intranasally. Her oxygen saturation was 97% on oxygen at 1400 hours Fluid restriction: 1 litre, strict FBC Daily weigh IVC in situ, prescribed IV frusemide. She has voided a total of 800 mLs this shift.
Referrals or reviews	Mr Samuel is going to review her this evening.

TABLE 10.5 Overview of therapeutic communication skills and relationships

Therapeutic relationship skills		**The four major therapeutic communication skills**			
Self-awareness	*Awareness of special situations*	*1. Listening*	*2. Understanding*	*3. Exploring*	*4. Psychosocial nursing actions*
Personal and professional development Processes: • introspection • input from others • self-sharing Areas of self-exploration: • health philosophy • values and beliefs • expectations of nursing Personal qualities and traits: • authenticity and congruence • respect and warmth • confidence and assertiveness	Transcultural communication Developmental stages: children and older adults Clients with communication difficulties Clients in stressful situations Clients in crisis	Effective active listening skills: • readiness • receptivity • attending • 'nursing' listening • observational skills • perceiving messages • interpreting (listening for themes) • recalling messages Barriers to active listening: • preoccupation • personal insecurity (e.g. anxiety) • unusual speech patterns/behaviours • physical discomfort • pychological discomfort (e.g. emotionality) • information 'overload'	Types of verbal responses: • advising and evaluating • analysing and interpreting • reassuring and supporting • questioning and probing • paraphrasing and understanding Therapeutic listening response skills: • minimal cues • clarification • restatement • paraphrasing • reflection • summarising • silence • touch Verbal response skills: • mirroring depth • matching response with verbal content	Asking questions Prompting questions: • minimal encouragement • one word/phrase accents • gentle commands • open-ended statements • starting (finishing) the sentence • self-disclosure Probing questions: • open-ended questions • focused open-ended questions • closed-ended questions • focused closed-ended questions • multiple-choice questions • follow-up questions	Comforting: • client's need for reassurance • nursing therapeutic communication skills • ideal outcomes Supporting: • client's need for support • nursing therapeutic communication skills • ideal outcomes Enabling: • client's need for enabling • nursing therapeutic communication skills (information/ education, challenging, self-disclosure) • ideal outcomes

TABLE 10.5 Overview of therapeutic communication skills and relationships—*cont'd*

Therapeutic relationship skills		**The four major therapeutic communication skills**			
Self-awareness	*Awareness of special situations*	*1. Listening*	*2. Understanding*	*3. Exploring*	*4. Psychosocial nursing actions*
			• appropriate language • focusing • using metaphors • reframing situations • presenting reality • using humour • confirming responses • giving feedback • asking for validation • anticipatory guidance	Cues from clients: • recognition of cues from clients • responding to cues from clients	

Source: Adapted from Arnold 2007, Stein-Parbury 2005.

? **QUESTION FOR REFLECTION**

Consider the areas for self-exploration listed in Table 10.5 under the column titled 'self-awareness'. What is your personal health philosophy? What are your key values and beliefs? What are your expectations of nursing?

Improving your verbal communication

It takes time and practice to become competent at verbal communication. For international nurses, this often seems overwhelming, as it requires both general English and 'nursing' English, as well as a sound understanding of medical terminology, jargon and abbreviations. It is important to remember that being proficient in English language is essential to being competent in verbal communication.

Review the strategies for improving your English (in Ch 2), and particularly focus on the strategies for developing your formal professional 'nursing' English listening and speaking skills (in Table 2.1). You are strongly encouraged to listen to nurses having conversations (on television programs and in clinical settings), to regularly update your 'Language list' (R2) (on the CD Part 3—Reader resources), to practise nursing conversations and handovers, and to ask a teacher or colleague to listen to you practise nursing conversations and handovers during clinical placements.

CHAPTER HIGHLIGHTS

- Verbal communication is an essential skill in nursing and is a core competency requirement for Australian and New Zealand nurses.
- Verbal communication is important for communicating patient information and for developing and maintaining relationships with patients and colleagues.
- The principles that guide verbal communication reflect the importance of communication in healthcare and the legal requirements for privacy and confidentiality of health information.
- To be effective in verbal communication, nurses need to be aware of the key aspects of verbal and non-verbal communication.
- Nurses use verbal communication in a variety of clinical situations.
- Nursing handover is widely used in clinical settings and is important for communicating information about patients, for staff debriefing and education.
- Therapeutic communication is a specialised application of advanced communication skills, and is directed towards promoting healing.
- Developing competency in verbal communication requires time and dedicated practice.

Self-test questions

1. Discuss the purposes of verbal communication in healthcare.
2. Describe the principles of verbal communication.
3. Outline the key aspects of verbal and non-verbal communication (and provide examples of how nurses can be effective at using verbal communication).

4. Listen to the CD Part 1—Audio, 'Nursing conversations' (A4–A14). Complete the 'Nursing conversations' activities and the self-test questions in Part 7.
5. Complete the 'Admission interview self-directed learning package' (R8) on the CD Part 3—Reader resources.
6. Complete the 'Mobilising and positioning patients self-directed learning package' (R9) on the CD Part 3—Reader resources.
7. Describe the types, purposes and formats of nursing handovers.
8. Read and summarise a recent journal article about nursing handover using the 'Article summary sheet' (R1) on the CD Part 3—Reader resources.
9. Listen to the CD Part 1—Audio, 'Nursing handovers' (A15–A16). Complete the 'Nursing handovers' activities and the self-test questions in Part 7.
10. Outline the four major skills required for therapeutic communication and provide a clinical example for each.
11. Review the key terms and any other new vocabulary, terms and abbreviations from this chapter, and then update your 'Language list' (R2) on the CD Part 3—Reader resources.
12. Answer the 'Learning objectives' at the start of this chapter as if they were examination questions.

References

Antai-Otong D 2006 Nurse–client communication. Elsevier, Sydney

Arnold EC 2007 Developing therapeutic communication skills in the nurse–client relationship. In: Arnold EC, Boggs KU (eds) 2007 Interpersonal relationships: professional communication skills for nurses, 5th edn. Elsevier, St Louis, pp 199–228

Chan C 2001 Moving with the times: the new handover—a change of practice (online). In: Smith J, Smith L, James P (eds) HIC 2001: proceedings, pp 215–24. Online. Available http://search.informit.com.au/documentSummary;dn=912703924078049;res=E-LIBRARY 12 Dec 2007

Dowd T, Eckermann K, Jeffs L 2009 Culture and ethnicity. In: Crisp J, Taylor C (eds) Potter & Perry's fundamentals of nursing, 3rd edn. Elsevier, Sydney, Ch 8

Gordon M 2006 Manual of nursing diagnosis, 11th edn. Jones & Bartlett, Boston

Levett-Jones T, Bourgeois S 2007 The clinical placement: an essential guide for nursing students. Elsevier, Sydney

Stein-Parbury J 2005 Patient and person: developing interpersonal skills in nursing, 3rd edn. Elsevier, Sydney

Stein-Parbury J 2009 Communication. In Crisp J, Taylor C (eds) Potter & Perry's fundamentals of nursing, 3rd edn. Elsevier, Sydney, Ch 23

Walton, J, Marriott R 2008 Culturally competent care. In: Brown D, Edwards H (eds) Lewis's medical–surgical nursing: assessment and management of clinical problems, 2nd edn. Elsevier, Sydney, pp 22–34

Recommended reading

New South Wales Health 2004 Communicating positively: a guide to appropriate Aboriginal terminology. Online. Available www.health.nsw.gov.au/pubs/ 2004/pdf/ ab_terminology. pdf 5 Mar 2008

Stein-Parbury J 2009 Communication. In Crisp J, Taylor C (eds) Potter & Perry's fundamentals of nursing, 3rd edn. Elsevier, Sydney, Ch 23

CHAPTER 11

Documentation

'Nurses must be very good at writing in the medical documents, and using the right abbreviations is very important. This is important so we can be legal and professional.'

Tak, Taiwan

CHAPTER OUTLINE

LEARNING OBJECTIVES

1. Discuss the purposes of documentation.
2. Discuss the principles of documentation.
3. Describe the types of documentation used in clinical nursing practice.
4. Describe in detail the legal implications associated with documentation.
5. Describe the styles of writing used in nursing documentation.
6. Demonstrate skills in 'nursing writing'.
7. Describe strategies to improve documentation skills.
8. Develop a personal plan for developing English language skills.

Key terms (are in bold in the text)

accountability
case management/case mix
clinical/critical pathways
continuity of care
DAR notes (focus charting)
demographic data
diagnostic related groups (DRG)
documentation
documenting by exception
focus charting (DAR notes)
multidisciplinary
narrative writing
nursing care plan (NCP)
nursing process
'nursing writing'
PIE (notes)
SOAPIE (notes)
24-hour clock/24-hour time
variances
(See also the types of documents listed in Table 11.1.)

Nursing students and graduate nurses often find documentation in clinical nursing settings to be a complex skill. A sound understanding of the purpose, principles and legal implications of documentation is required, along with familiarity with the types of documents used for recording patient or client information. In addition, all nurses need to develop skills in the styles of writing used for documenting in clinical settings.

Documentation: principles and practices

It is a nursing competency requirement that you can communicate effectively in English. To be a safe and competent nurse and nursing student, you *must* be able to demonstrate excellent written communication or documentation skills. (See Ch 5 for a detailed discussion of nursing competency standards.)

Purpose of documentation

The key purposes of **documentation** in healthcare are to meet legal requirements, to communicate information to ensure continuity of care for the patient or client, to serve as a record of the contribution by various disciplines (of health professionals) to the care of the patient or client (Astell & Bourke 2009 Ch 25, Axford in Schulz-Robinson 1997 p 174), and to facilitate quality management, research and funding (Astell & Bourke 2009 Ch 25).

Legal requirement

Documentation is a skill required of all health professionals (Fitzgerald 2008 pp 13–14, Jamieson 1997, Levett-Jones & Bourgeois 2007 p 103), and is 'an integral part of the nurse's legal obligation to both employer and client' (Jamieson 1997 p 63).

Communication

The various documents used in healthcare settings provide considerable information about patients or clients. These documents detail their **demographic data**, health history, family (medical) history, allergies, ongoing health conditions and treatments (including medication use), current condition, problems and diagnosis, current treatment and planned care, including referrals and discharge plans.

Continuity of care is a term used to reflect the ongoing nature of patient or client care (even when the care is delivered intermittently—such as in a community or clinic setting—and not continuously as occurs when a person is hospitalised or lives in a residential care facility). By maintaining accurate records, a person's care can continue from shift to shift or even from one consultation with a health professional to another.

When the planned or actual care provided is documented clearly, it can be continued; hence, 'continuity of care' is maintained.

Contribution to care by various disciplines

When documenting patient or client care, health professionals—including nurses—are also documenting what they do. It is important to note, however, that nursing documentation is not simply a list of tasks that the nurse has completed. Nursing documentation should be patient or client focused, but it will be written from a nurse's perspective and will inevitably also record what nursing care the nurse has provided. Therefore, nursing documentation reflects nursing and can illuminate nursing. Schulz-Robinson argues 'the work of nurses is defined by what they document' (1997 p 173). For these reasons, reviews of nursing documentation have been used as a method of researching nursing and developing nursing theories (particularly when considering the questions 'what is nursing?' and 'what do nurses do?').

From a legal perspective, documentation also 'reflects the quality of the care and provides evidence of each healthcare team member's **accountability** in the delivery of the care' (Astell & Bourke 2009 Ch 25). This is particularly important in **multidisciplinary** care models, where a number of health professionals from various disciplines care for a client or patient.

Quality management, research and funding

Reviews of documentation provide information for quality management (this might be related to the documentation itself or to clinical care issues). Documentation also provides valuable audit data, statistics and information for research purposes. In some situations, hospital funding (from the government) is calculated according to the types of 'cases' it treats. This is referred to as the **case mix** or **case management** model, which originated in the United States, whereby **diagnostic related groups (DRGs)** are developed according to the patient's diagnosis, history, procedures and age, and the hospital is reimbursed according to the DRG.

A very simplified example would be where a hospital is reimbursed a set amount for the patients admitted for total hip replacement surgery. Documentation of the care required for the patients having this type of surgery provides evidence for developing—or modifying—the DRG and costing it (Astell & Bourke 2009 Ch 25).

Types of documents

The types of documents used to record patient or client information in healthcare settings will vary slightly according to the facility, and it is important to be familiar with the types of documents you will be using. It is also necessary to be familiar with the various terminology, jargon and abbreviations used to describe these documents. This varies, but remember to use the abbreviations and terminology accepted in the facility where you are working or doing a clinical placement. Table 11.1 describes the types of documents used in healthcare settings. Documents are provided in 'Sample hospital documents' (R13) on the CD Part 3—Reader resources.

TABLE 11.1 Description of healthcare documents

Type of document	Description	Written by:	Location	Nursing implications
Medical record/patient history/the history/patient file/the file/ patient notes/the notes (the specific types of documents in the patient file are listed separately in this table—in the 'Location' column, 'patient file' is noted)	A *set* of documents containing many separate documents about a particular patient or client (including notes written by health professionals, test results, reports of operations or procedures, and the set of documents that make up the files of previous admissions to the same facility)	All health professionals (varies according to each document)	Binder or folder (stored away from the bedside in hospital settings)	All the information in the patient file must remain private and confidential
Bedside charts/patient charts (the specific types of bedside charts are listed separately in this table—in the 'Location' column, 'bedside charts' is noted)	A *set* of documents containing a number of separate documents that are updated frequently (including drug charts, IV orders, vital signs chart)	Nurses and medical practitioners (doctors), depending on the document	Binder, folder or clipboard, usually stored at/near the bedside (in hospital settings)	All the information in the patient file must remain private and confidential
Nursing admission form/nursing admission interview form/nursing admission and health history form	A form or sheet for documenting information about the patient from the admission interview	Nurses	Patient file	
Progress notes	A form or sheet for documenting information about the patient on a regular basis (i.e. each shift in acute settings, daily in subacute settings or at set intervals—for example, 7th day of each month in residential settings)	Integrated progress notes—all health professionals (always in chronological order, with the discipline noted at the start of the entry) Separate progress notes—discipline specific (e.g. nursing, medical, allied health sections)	Patient file	Commence all nursing entries with the word 'Nursing:'

(Continued)

TABLE 11.1 Description of healthcare documents—*cont'd*

Type of document	Description	Written by:	Location	Nursing implications
Medical notes/medical orders (in 'progress notes')	A form or sheet for documenting information about the medical assessment and medical care (including orders for other health professionals)	Medical practitioner (doctor)	Patient file—usually in the 'progress notes' section if the notes from all disciplines are integrated (or in the 'medical progress notes' section if the discipline notes are separate)	
Nursing notes/notes (in the 'progress notes')	A form or sheet for documenting information about the nursing assessment and nursing care of the patient	Nurses	Patient file—usually in the 'progress notes' section if the notes from all disciplines are integrated (or in the 'nursing progress notes' section if the discipline notes are separate)	Commence all entries with the word 'Nursing:' 'Nursing progress notes' include: • 'nursing notes', which document every shift or daily (shift/daily) notes, and document the patient's condition and nursing care (notes may also be about preoperative care, postoperative care or an incident) • 'admission notes', which are documented on admission, and document the patient's PHx, current Dx, condition and planned care • 'discharge notes', which are documented on discharge, and document the patient's discharge, condition and planned ongoing care

TABLE 11.1 Description of healthcare documents—*cont'd*

Type of document	Description	Written by:	Location	Nursing implications
Clinical pathways/critical pathways	A chart outlining the expected progress and care required for the patient based on the medical diagnosis. Lists all care and due date for all health professionals (e.g. clinical pathway for patient having total knee replacement or clinical pathway for patient with COPD). This is a multidisciplinary document	All health professionals involved in the care of the patient (multidisciplinary)	Patient file or bedside charts	Variances from the expected progress in the pathway (arising from any complications) are recorded either on the variance section of the pathway document or in the progress notes
Nursing care plan (NCP)	A chart for recording the patient problems and nursing care to be provided (has columns or sections for problems, goals, care and evaluation)	Nurses	Patient file or bedside charts	Some facilities use pre-printed NCPs and the nurses add to them as required
Vital signs chart/observations chart ('obs' chart)/TPR chart/thermic chart	A chart for recording TPR, BP and weight, urinalysis results and bowel actions	Nurses	Bedside charts	
Fluid balance chart (FBC)	A chart for recording the patient's fluid intake and output over a 24-hour period	Nurse	Bedside charts	
Fluid balance summary	A chart for recording the 24-hour fluid total intake and output (from the FBC)	Nurse	Bedside charts	
Special observation or assessment charts (e.g. blood sugar level (BSL) or blood glucose level (BGL) chart, faecal description chart (FDC) and food chart)	A chart for recording specific assessments	Nurse	Bedside charts	

(Continued)

TABLE 11.1 Description of healthcare documents—*cont'd*

Type of document	Description	Written by:	Location	Nursing implications
Drug chart/drug orders chart/ medication chart ('med' chart)/medication sheet	A chart for documenting the drugs/ medications prescribed for the patient and the administration of the drugs/medications (there are various types—some are drug-specific; some include IV fluid orders; and some have separate sections for injectable drugs, subcutaneous or IV drugs, telephone orders, nurse-initiated drugs)	Prescription (or orders)—medical practitioner (doctor) Administration—nurse or doctor (who administers the drug)	Bedside charts or patient file (or in a separate drug charts folder in some residential settings)	Administration is indicated by initialling the correct space (for the drug, date and time) Use *only* abbreviations accepted at the facility for indicating refusal by the patient or inability to administer the drug
IV chart/IV fluids chart/IV orders	A chart for documenting the IV fluids prescribed for the patient and the administration of the IV fluids	Prescription (or orders)—medical practitioner (doctor) Administration—nurse or doctor (who administers the IV fluids)	Bedside charts or patient file	Two RNs (or RNs Div 1) need to sign the administration of narcotics and IV fluid
Preoperative ('pre-op') checklist	Sheet with provision for ticking items to be attended before sending a patient for surgery. It often lists the documents to include in the 'patient file' (e.g. completed consent form, blank anaesthetic record, blank operation report, current drug chart) and activities to perform, such as check ID label in situ, record allergies, sign pre-medication order if administered)	Nurse	Patient file (often attached to the outside front cover)	Discarded after the operation (as this is a checklist and not part of the patient medical record)
Postoperative observation chart ('post-op obs chart)	A chart for recording postoperative vital signs and other assessments	Nurse	Bedside charts during postoperative recovery period and then filed in patient file	

TABLE 11.1 Description of healthcare documents—*cont'd*

Type of document	Description	Written by:	Location	Nursing implications
Procedure report/operation report	Sheets or pages for documenting the event (e.g. gastroscopy)	Medical practitioner (specialist) who performed the procedure	Patient file	
Anaesthetic record	Sheets or pages for documenting the event (includes sections for preoperative assessment by anaesthetist, pre-medication orders, listing the anaesthetic drugs administered, vital signs during anaesthetic and recovery)	Anaesthetist and anaesthetic nurse	Patient file	
Diagnostic report	Sheets or pages for documenting the results (e.g. of blood tests) or findings (e.g. report of X-ray; report about a tissue sample removed in a biopsy) of tests/procedures/operations	Medical practitioner (specialist) who is responsible for reporting the diagnostic findings (e.g. a radiologist reports on X-rays)	Patient file	
Referral	A document for referring the patient to another health professional (within a hospital, a referral sheet is used; for external referrals, a letter is usually written)	Referring health professional (i.e. the one who is referring the patient)	Copy retained in patient file	
Discharge summary	A sheet or form for documenting a summary of the patient's hospital stay and ongoing care needs Copy usually provided to patient's community-based carers (e.g. GP, community nurse) or residential care service	Medical practitioner or nurse	Copy retained in patient file	

(Continued)

TABLE 11.1 Description of healthcare documents—*cont'd*

Type of document	Description	Written by:	Location	Nursing implications
Consent form	A sheet signed by the patient and medical practitioner to verify that the patient consents (agrees) to a procedure or operation	Patient and medical practitioner *only*	Patient file	Nurses should *never* sign a consent form (even as a witness) and most facilities have a policy about this
Incident report	A document for recording an unexpected or unusual event or accident (e.g. patient fall, drug administration error, needlestick injury) Some incident reports are general (and used for all types of incidents) Some incident reports are specific and used only for the type of incident specified (e.g. falls incident report or drug error incident report)	Witness, nurse and medical practitioner, and designated senior hospital medical and nursing staff (e.g. director of medicine, director of nursing)	Patient file	Incident reports *must* be clear, accurate and objective. Incident reports are a record of the incident, *not* an admission of guilt or a statement of blame Incident reports are an important part of healthcare risk management and quality management systems at a facility

Legal implications of documentation

It is critical to remember that 'all medical and nursing records are potential legal documents' (Jamieson 1997 p 63) and that 'documentation is considered to be the most important evidence in a potential legal action' (Levett-Jones & Bourgeois 2007 p 103).

If your documentation is examined in a legal case, remember that it will most likely be many years after you have written it. It is also likely that it will be your only aid to recalling the specific care you provided. If your notes are not sufficiently accurate, factual, objective, complete or clear, you will have difficulty providing evidence of the care you provided. When writing about the care you provide, remember the saying 'not documented, not done' (Mandell 1994), which means that if you do not document your nursing care, it will be assumed that you did not provide the care.

QUESTION FOR REFLECTION

Read the scenarios in Boxes 11.1 and 11.2, and consider which examples are most like the nursing notes you currently write.

Box 11.1 Scenario 1—Patient with permanent left hand nerve damage related to compartment syndrome

Notes A
Patient reported L hand pain. Dr paged.

Notes B
At 1600 hr patient reported pain in left hand, described as crushing, rating 10/10 on a pain scale. POP in situ to L forearm. L hand neurovascular assessment: L fingers pale, cool to touch, patient unable to move fingers, sensation diminished in all digits, capillary return greater than 3 secs, radial pulse unable to be assessed due to POP, reports 'severe' pain on passive movement. R hand neurovascular assessment: pink, warm to touch, movement and sensation present, nil pain reported, radial pulse palpable 96 bpm, capillary return less than 1 sec. Dr Brown notified via pager at 1610 hr and reviewed patient at 1620 hr. POP removed by Dr Brown.

Court case allegation: The patient sues the hospital for the damage to his left hand.
Date: 5 years later.
Question you are asked: What did you do about the patient's left hand pain?

If you had written Notes A, you would not have sufficient written evidence of your nursing care. If you had written Notes B, you would have a detailed record of the assessment you made, and of the action you took.

Principles of documentation

The principles of documentation relate primarily to the legal requirements associated with recording healthcare information. To ensure that your documentation satisfies these legal requirements, you will need to be able to document in a manner that meets the key principles and writing conventions detailed in Table 11.2.

Box 11.2 Scenario 2—Patient who sustained a head injury from a fall out of bed

Notes A
Patient RIB after admission.

Notes B
Patient falls risk assessment conducted as charted. Patient advised to remain RIB and not to attempt to ambulate without nursing staff present. Patient's daughter (Ms Scott) present during admission and advised of same. Demonstrated use of call bell and call bell pinned to patient's pillow. Patient able to demonstrate correct use of call bell. Cot sides in situ. Patient alert and orientated.

Court case allegation: The patient's family claim nursing staff were negligent with respect to the patient's injury.
Date: 3 years later.
Question you are asked: Describe what you did to reduce the risk of injury and promote the patient's safety.

If you had written Notes A, you would not have sufficient written evidence of the care you provided. If you had written Notes B, you would have a detailed record of the risk assessment, risk management and patient education you provided.

The 24-hour clock

The **24-hour clock**, also known as **24 time**, is used extensively in healthcare, and you must be able to use this style in verbal and written communication (see Figs 11.1, 11.2 and 11.3). (Listen to the CD Part 1—Audio, 'Nursing handovers' (A15–A16).) The examples in Table 11.3 have key points to note in italics.

FIGURE 11.1 The 24-hour clock

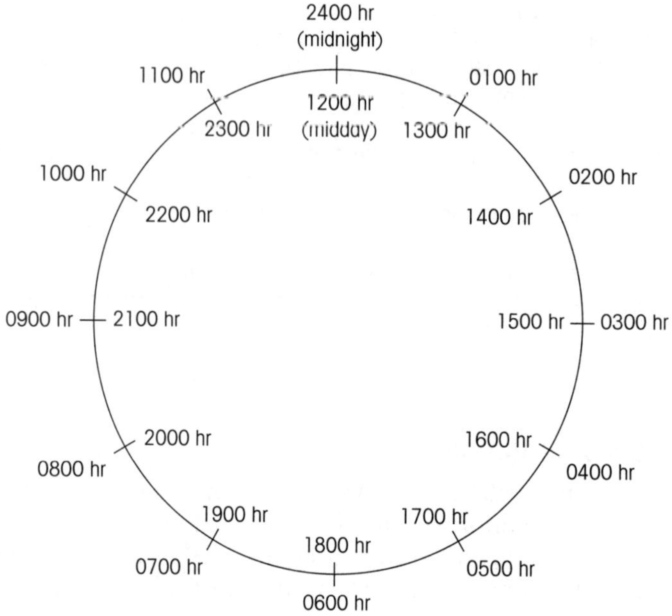

FIGURE 11.2 Standard and 24-hour times: a.m.

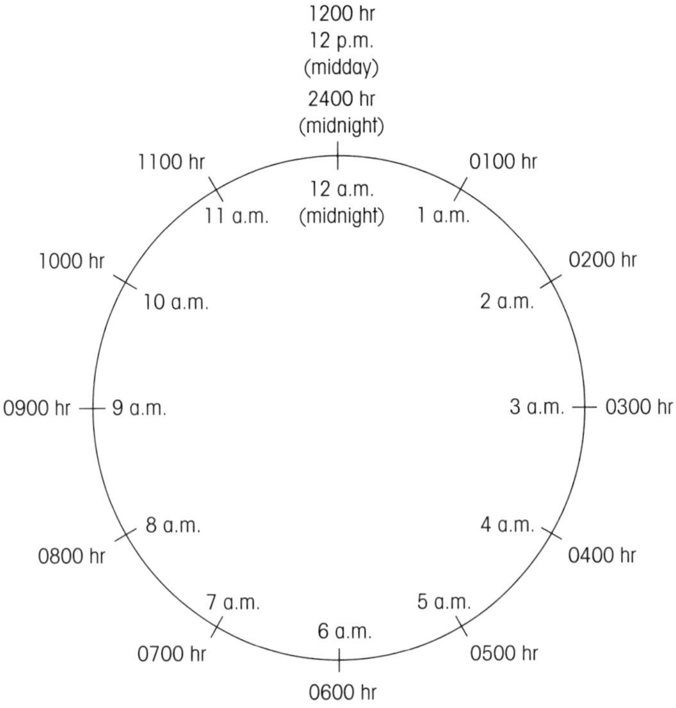

FIGURE 11.3 Standard and 24-hour times: p.m.

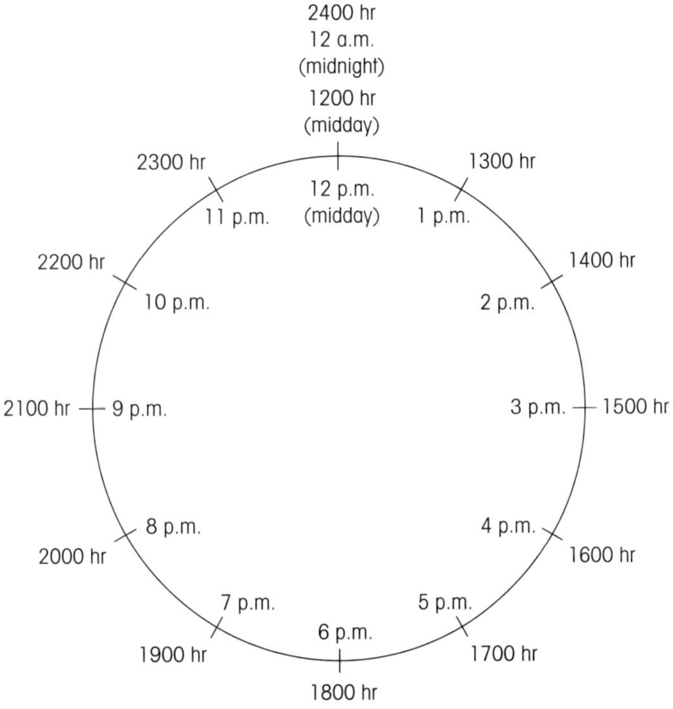

TABLE 11.2 Legal principles and conventions of documentation

Legal principles		
Principle	*Explanation/rationale*	*Examples*
Accurate	Be specific and correct.	At 1400 hr pt c/o feeling 'dizzy' while RIB. BP 85/55 mmHg at 1400 hr. Dr Hammersly notified and reviewed pt. At 1415 hr IV infusion rate increased as ordered. At 1430 hr BP 90/60 mmHg and pt reported dizziness has resolved. *Not*: Pt had low BP. [This is not specific, accurate or sufficiently factual. It is incomplete, as it does not document the assessment, intervention or evaluation.]
Factual	Be truthful.	
Objective	Avoid subjective comments or personal opinions.	
Complete	Avoid omissions (do not leave out important information, including nursing assessments, interventions or evaluations, or patient education or advice). If care is omitted, document why.	Pt c/o RLQ abdominal pain, described as 'dull and cramping' rating 9/10 on pain scale. *Not*: Pt has severe abdominal pain. [This is not objective or sufficiently accurate. It is incomplete, as it does not document the assessment.] Pt is pale, diaphoretic and c/o feeling unwell. T 39C, P 102 irregular, R 24, BP 120/85, SaO2 92% on room air. *Not*: Pt seems very unwell. [This is not objective or sufficiently accurate. It is incomplete, as it does not document the assessment.] Dressing to sacral pressure sore attended as per NCP. Wound 5 cm in diameter, red, granulation tissue present, no slough. Nil c/o pain at site. *Not*: Wound dressing attended. [This is not objective or sufficiently accurate. It is incomplete, as it does not document the assessment.] Pt refused lactulose at 0800 hr, and stated she had diarrhoea x 5 overnight. Dr McKenna notified and aperient order changed to PRN. BNO this shift. *Not*: Refused lactulose. [This is not complete, as it does not document the assessment and nursing actions.]
Concise	Be brief. Avoid repetition and do not routinely repeat data or information recorded on other documents. Repeat only unusual or significant data in the progress notes. If the patient's pulse was rapid	Use a concise writing style. For narrative notes, use 'nursing writing'. Do not write 'at 1200 hr the patient consumed 200 mL of fluid' in the nursing progress notes if it is documented on the FBC.

TABLE 11.2 Legal principles and conventions of documentation—*cont'd*

Legal principles		
Principle	*Explanation/rationale*	*Examples*
Concise—*cont'd*	and irregular and was reported to the doctor, and required intervention, this should be documented in both the nursing progress notes and the vital signs chart.	
Contemporaneous (i.e. timely)	Document assessment data at the time it is measured. Document incidents or unexpected changes as they occur. Progress notes can be written at the end of the shift, with the date and time of writing noted. Identify late entries.	When measuring vital signs, record them immediately. If a patient becomes unwell, record the assessment, management and evaluation of the situation at the time it occurs. For example: 14/4/08 1500 hr NURSING: . . . For example: 21/4/08 0730 hr NURSING Late entry for 20/4/08: . . .
Privacy and confidentiality	Nurses must ensure that documents containing patient information remain private and confidential, according to the laws governing privacy and confidentiality of health information. Secure document storage, and access to documents only by relevant and appropriate health professionals (involved in the patient's care) and protection of the information contained in the documents (limited to health professionals involved in the patient's care, the patient or with the patient's consent significant others) are nursing responsibilities.	
Document only for yourself	*Never* document information (e.g. vital signs) or sign (e.g. drug administration) for another person. You are accountable for both your actions and the information you document.	

(Continued)

TABLE 11.2 Legal principles and conventions of documentation—*cont'd*

Conventions		
Convention	*Explanation/rationale*	*Examples*
Always check that the information is documented in the correct patient's file.	Documenting in the incorrect file could have very serious consequences for patient care and also have legal ramifications.	
Legible writing	Documentation must be able to be read.	
Ink, not pencil	Ink cannot be altered easily, unlike pencil.	
Avoid erasures and deletion ('white-out') products.	Attempts to change entries could be misinterpreted as falsifying records. If an error is made, draw a single line through it and initial above the line.	Pt reported feeling ~~constipated~~ [JK] nauseated.
Avoid spaces on charts and in notes.	Complete the next available line or section of charts. Use a line instead of leaving a space in progress notes. This prevents alterations to your notes by others.	Pt RIB. Nil c/o abdominal pain this shift. HNPU since RTW.
Use only accepted abbreviations (as per facility policy).	Abbreviations could have multiple meanings and the use of your own personal abbreviations could make documentation unclear.	
Commence entries with the date and time, and in progress notes note the discipline.	Date must be written in the following order: day/month/year or day.month.year. Time must be written using the 24-hour clock.	10/8/08 2100 hr NURSING 21.7.08 1630 hr NURSING
At the end of entries, sign and print your name in English,	The person signing the documentation is accountable for the information recorded.	S/B Dr Irving. For r/v by Mr Raywood after CXR tomorrow afternoon. *S.Cheng*. S. Cheng BN student (Greenacres Uni) *J. Kenburg*. J.Kenburg RN

TABLE 11.2 Legal principles and conventions of documentation—*cont'd*

Conventions		
Convention	*Explanation/rationale*	*Examples*
using the initial of your given name and your full family name (surname).	English characters *must* be used.	
Note designation using accepted abbreviations.	Note that all student nurse entries *must* be countersigned by an RN. Use an accepted abbreviation for 'student nurse' and note the institution where you are enrolled.	

Sources: Astell & Bourke 2005 pp 472–5, Jamieson 1997 p 64, Levett-Jones & Bourgeois 2007 pp 103–7, Mandell 1994.

TABLE 11.3 Examples of 24-hour time

Standard time		**Twenty-four hour time**	
Written	***Verbal***	***Written***	***Verbal***
6 p.m.	Six p.m. Six o'clock in the evening	1800 hr	Eighteen hundred hours
8.30 a.m.	Eight thirty a.m. Half past eight in the morning	0830 hr	Zero eight thirty hours *O eight thirty hours**
9.10 a.m.	Nine ten a.m. Ten past nine in the morning	0910 hr	Zero nine ten hours O nine ten hours*
11.55 p.m.	Eleven fifty-five p.m. Five to twelve at night Five to midnight	2355 hr	Twenty-three fifty-five hours
11.45 a.m.	Eleven forty-five a.m. *A quarter to twelve in the morning* (morning refers to the time, not 'twelve in the morning', which is midnight)	1145 hr	Eleven forty-five hours
12 a.m.	Midnight Twelve a.m.	2400 hr	Twenty-four hundred hours
12.15 a.m.	Twelve fifteen a.m. *A quarter past twelve in the morning*** *A quarter past midnight***	0015 hr (*not* 2415 hr)***	*Zero zero fifteen hours (not twenty-four fifteen hours)*
12 p.m.	Midday Twelve p.m.	1200 hr	Twelve hundred hours
12.15 p.m.	Twelve fifteen p.m. *A quarter past twelve in the afternoon*** *A quarter past midday***	1215 hr	Twelve fifteen hours

*In Australia and New Zealand, people often say (the letter) O instead of (the number) zero. While this is not grammatically correct, it is very common in spoken English.

**Fifteen minutes to or fifteen minutes past the hour is expressed in standard time as 'a quarter to' or 'a quarter past' the hour (as in a quarter of an hour, which is 15 minutes) and never as 'fifteen past' or 'fifteen to'.

***Midnight is 2400 hr. All time past midnight is recorded using 00, not 24 (i.e. 0005 hr, 0030 hr, 0055 hr).

Writing in nursing practice

Nurses need to be proficient at documenting in various ways. Documenting some assessments and measurements is often straightforward, as numeric data is usually recorded on charts (e.g. vital signs charts, FBCs). When tick sheets or checklists are used (e.g. preoperative checklist, clinical/critical pathways), there is also little writing required. Assessment documents or forms (e.g. nursing admission form, pressure area

TABLE 11.4 Comparing English writing and 'nursing writing'

	English writing	'Nursing writing'
Sentences	Full sentences	Short sentences
Abbreviations	Not used	Used appropriately
Medical terminology	Not generally used	Used appropriately
Examples	The patient has a past history of breast cancer.	(Pt has) PHx Ca breast
	At 10 p.m., Mr Jones reported that he had chest pain.	At 2200 hr pt c/o PIC
	Mrs Smith sat out of bed for half an hour.	(Pt) SOOB for 30/60

risk assessment form) usually have a questionnaire format and require relatively little writing, although the correct use of abbreviations is required. Nursing progress notes, referrals and letters, however, usually require a style of writing that requires practice for nurses to master.

Documenting styles

Narrative writing

There are many methods for organising narrative (or story-telling) writing. Essentially, the patient's problems, nursing assessments, interventions and evaluations need to be documented. This is consistent with the **nursing process** (discussed in Ch 13) and some facilities use the nursing care plan, or an assessment framework, such as Gordon's functional health patterns (see Box 10.1) or the body systems as the basis for nursing notes. This is referred to as problem-based or problem-oriented notes. These notes can be written in a number of formats including **SOAPIE** (Subjective data, Objective data, Assessment and nursing diagnosis, Plan of care, Interventions or nursing care, Evaluation of care), **PIE** (Problem, Intervention, Evaluation) or **focus charting**, also known as **DAR notes** (Data, Action or nursing care, Response or evaluation).

Documenting by exception

Documenting by exception requires the use of a document such as a detailed nursing care plan or a clinical/critical pathway that clearly states the standard care for the patient. The nurse then documents only variations from the standard care outlined in the nursing care plan or clinical/critical pathway (using a narrative method). This style requires that the nursing care plan is regularly updated and usually the nurse must sign that care has been provided or state 'care provided as per NCP', remembering that if the care is not documented it is not considered to have been provided.

Documenting in nursing care plans

The **nursing care plan (NCP)** is a nursing document developed and used by nurses to record the nursing care planned for the patient. In general, the nurse writes an individualised NCP based on assessment of the patient. Some facilities use standardised NCPs to which the nurse adds individualised information relevant for the particular patient.

All NCPs should specify the patient problems (nursing diagnosis), goals, plans and interventions, along with expected evaluation information.

Documenting in clinical/critical pathways

Clinical/critical pathways are essentially standardised multidisciplinary care plans outlining the expected progress and care required for the patient based on the medical diagnosis. The checklist format specifies the day, the care and the health professional responsible for the care, from admission to discharge. **Variances** (or changes from the expected pathway) must be documented on either the variance record, which is part of the clinical/critical pathway document, or in the progress notes (using a narrative method). This is also an example of documenting by exception.

Regardless of the documentation style used for nursing notes, all reports about the patient's condition made to medical practitioners and all clarification sought for medical orders (e.g. checking the dose of a drug prescribed) should be clearly documented.

'Nursing writing'

In this text, the term '**nursing writing**' is used to refer to the narrative style of writing used by nurses in nursing progress notes, nursing admission and discharge documents, and referral letters. In some cases, this style is also required for documenting in nursing care plans (particularly the interventions) and clinical/critical pathways (particularly in variance records). Table 11.4 provides some examples of 'nursing writing'.

Improving your documentation

It takes time and practice to become competent at documentation. For international nurses, documentation often seems overwhelming, as it requires both general English and 'nursing' English, as well as a sound understanding of medical terminology, jargon and abbreviations. It is important to remember that being proficient in English language is essential to being competent in documentation. Review the strategies for improving your English (in Ch 2), and focus on the strategies for developing your formal professional 'nursing' English reading and writing skills (in Table 2.1).

You are strongly encouraged to review documents (from 'Sample hospital documents' (R13) on the CD Part 3—Reader resources, other texts and clinical settings), read sample documentation (from textbooks) and actual documentation found in clinical settings and to regularly update your 'Language list' (R2) on the CD Part 3—Reader resources. It is also very important to practise 'nursing writing', using the 'Nursing documentation checklist' (R6.8) in the 'Clinical placement folio' (R6) on the CD Part 3—Reader resources, and to ask a teacher or colleague to review a draft of your progress notes and other documentation during clinical placements.

CHAPTER HIGHLIGHTS

- Documentation is an essential skill in nursing and is a core competency requirement for Australian and New Zealand nurses.

- Documentation is legally required in healthcare and is important for communicating patient information, reflecting the accountability of health professionals and for quality management, research and funding.
- Nurses must be able to document using a variety of types of documents.
- There are legal implications related to documentation and all health records can become legal documents.
- The principles and writing conventions that guide documentation are related to the legal implications associated with documentation.
- Nurses use different documentation styles to chart numeric data, complete tick sheets and checklists, complete questionnaires and write narrative notes.
- 'Nursing writing' is the style of writing used by nurses in narrative methods and differs from general English in that it is very concise, and abbreviations and medical terminology are used.
- Developing competency in documentation requires time and dedicated practice.

Self-test questions

1. Discuss the purposes of documentation in healthcare.
2. Using available resources (including 'Sample hospital documents' (R13) on the CD Part 3—Reader resources, other textbooks, samples from your teaching institution or *blank* samples from clinical settings that do *not* contain any confidential information, used with permission) obtain copies of the documents listed in Table 11.1.
3. Describe the information recorded on each of the documents listed in Table 11.1.
4. Discuss the legal implications related to documentation.
5. Describe your responsibilities in meeting the legal principles and writing conventions associated with healthcare documentation.
6. Briefly describe the terms 'narrative writing' and 'documenting by exception' as they relate to documenting in nursing.
7. Review the documents from the sources listed below:

   Sample NCP: Patient with COPD:

   Brown D, Edwards H (eds) 2008 Lewis's medical–surgical nursing: assessment and management of clinical problems, 2nd edn. Elsevier, Sydney, pp 708–10

   Sample clinical/critical pathway: elective total knee replacement (TKR) surgery:

   www.ciap.health.nsw.gov.au/hospolic/stvincents/1992/a03.html#a1

   Sample clinical/critical pathways: coronary artery bypass graft (CABG) surgery:

   Crisp J, Taylor C (eds) 2009 Potter & Perry's fundamentals of nursing, 3rd edn. Elsevier, Sydney, Ch 49

   Discuss the differences between nursing care plans and clinical/critical pathways.
8. Read and summarise a recent journal article about documentation in nursing using the 'Article summary sheet' (R1) on the CD Part 3—Reader resources.
9. Using the information obtained from your patient admission interview (from Ch 10, Self-test question 5), write a set of nursing progress notes using standard general English and then write a set of progress notes using 'nursing writing'. (Remember to follow the documentation principles and writing conventions.)

10. Review the key terms and any other new vocabulary, terms and abbreviations from this chapter, and then update your 'Language list' (R2) on the CD Part 3—Reader resources.

11. Answer the 'Learning objectives' at the start of this chapter as if they were examination questions.

References

Astell L, Bourke L 2009 Documentation. In: Crisp J, Taylor C (eds) Potter & Perry's fundamentals of nursing, 3rd edn. Elsevier, Sydney, Ch 25

Fitzgerald M 2008 The importance of nursing. In: Brown D, Edwards H (eds) Lewis's medical–surgical nursing: assessment and management of clinical problems, 2nd edn. Elsevier, Sydney, pp 2–21

Jamieson A 1997 Legal issues in documentation. In: Richmond J (ed) Nursing documentation: writing what we do. Ausmed, Melbourne, pp 63–70

Levett-Jones T, Bourgeois S 2007 The clinical placement: an essential guide for nursing students. Elsevier, Sydney

Mandell M 1994 Not documented, not done. Nursing 24(8):62

Schulz-Robinson S 1997 A political imperative: make nurses' work visible by documentation. In: Richmond J (ed) Nursing documentation: writing what we do. Ausmed, Melbourne, pp 173–9

PART 5

Clinical placement

CHAPTER 12

Preparing for clinical placement

'I think all students need to be very prepared for clinicals. This experience is very important.'

Olivia, Fiji

CHAPTER OUTLINE

LEARNING OBJECTIVES

1. Discuss the purposes of clinical placement.
2. Describe the types of schedules and settings for clinical placements.
3. Discuss the models for teaching, support and supervision of nursing students during clinical placements.
4. Identify the general requirements and expectations that educational institutions and clinical placement facilities have of nursing students with regard to clinical placements.
5. Discuss the learning requirements and expectations associated with clinical placements.
6. Develop a personal plan for preparing for clinical placements.

Key terms (are in bold in the text)

clinical agency
clinical education
clinical educators
clinical experience
clinical facilitators
clinical facility
clinical placement
clinical practicum
clinical supervisors
clinical teachers
competency assessment tool
competency standards
educational institutions
field experience
fieldwork
learning objectives
praxis
reflection
reflective practice

Almost every nursing student feels anxious about clinical placements. Clinical placements provide numerous challenges for students and unlimited opportunities for learning, and for personal and professional development. They can be particularly challenging for overseas nurses and international nursing students, because the clinical environment is a subculture, where healthcare beliefs, practices and language need to be understood.

To succeed in your clinical placements—and working in any clinical setting—in Australia or New Zealand, you will need to be well prepared. As part of your preparation, it is also strongly recommended that you read a text that addresses clinical placement issues, listed in the 'Recommended reading' (Levett-Jones & Bourgeois 2007).

Clinical placement

The **clinical placement** is also known as **clinical experience**, **clinical practice**, **field experience**, **fieldwork** and **clinical practicum**. It is the component of all nursing courses where students spend time in a real clinical setting.

Purposes

In a practice-based discipline such as nursing, **clinical education** is an essential component of all pre-registration—and many postgraduate—courses. The nursing regulatory authorities in Australia and New Zealand specifiy the minimum clinical placement requirements for all accredited courses offered by **educational institutions**.

Clinical placements provide students with the opportunity for **praxis**. This complex concept, long considered important in nursing, is most simply defined as the interaction of theory, research and practice (Rolfe 1993, 2006, Tarlier 2005). During clinical placements, students can apply theory to practice, further expand their theoretical knowledge, perform clinical skills and apply clinical knowledge to theoretical concepts.

Clinical placement also provides the opportunity for **reflection** or **reflective practice** (Levett-Jones & Bourgeois 2007 pp 116–21). Reflection is defined in numerous ways in the nursing literature (Bulman 2004 pp 2–4), but essentially requires 'the exploration of an experience, the analysis of feelings or of self to inform learning'(Bulman 2004 p 4). It has the potential to lead to a 'changed perspective and action' (Bulman 2004 p 4). While there is some debate about how nurses use reflection (Alliex & McCarthy 2005), it is a practice included in the curricula of Australia and New Zealand nursing courses and is also a specific requirement as stated in the competency standards for nurses in both countries (Australian Nursing and Midwifery Council 2002, 2006, Nursing Council of New Zealand 2007a, 2007b).

Schedules

Clinical placement scheduling occurs in a variety of ways. Sometimes, clinical placements occur intermittently (e.g. 2 days each week over 6 weeks), and at other times 'blocks' are arranged (e.g. a 2-week period).

Settings

Clinical placements take place in many settings, and are arranged so students can maximise their learning opportunities in a broad range of areas. Nursing students attend placements in the public and private healthcare sectors, in hospitals, aged care facilities, community organisations, in government facilities and in private companies. Clinical placements can be arranged in urban, rural and remotes areas. Students are provided with a range of clincal placements to provide them with acute, subacute, community, forensic, adult, aged care, adolescent, paediatric and nursing specialty area experiences. The place where the placement occurs is referred to as the **clinical facility** or **clinical agency**.

Models for teaching, supervision and support

The nursing regulatory authorities in Australia and New Zealand require that suitable registered nurses supervise students at all times during all clinical placements. Table 12.1 describes the models for teaching, supervision and support during clinical placement. It should be noted that although the terminology can vary in different contexts—with mentoring usually referring to a process that enhances one's career opportunities and prospects (Mills et al 2003)—the terms used here relate to nursing student clinical placements in Australia and New Zealand.

While facility staff contribute to the clinical education of nursing students, through 'buddying' and mentoring, the educational institution is responsible for employing and providing **clinical teachers** (also called **clinical educators**, **clinical facilitators** or **clinical supervisors**), or training and supporting facility-based **preceptors**. This is because the relevant nursing regulatory authority accredits educational institutions to provide courses that include theoretical and practical components within their curriculum.

Before starting a clinical placement, you should know the type of supervision that will be provided.

Preparation for clinical placement

Preparation for clinical placement should occur before the clinical placement. This will greatly reduce the stress that students often experience at the start of a clinical placement. Use the 'Clinical placement preparation checklist' (R6.1), in the 'Clinical placement folio' (R6) on the CD Part 3—Reader resources, to assist you to prepare for your clinical placements.

TABLE 12.1 Models for teaching, supervision and support during clinical placement

Type of supervisor	Employed by:	Key roles and responsibilities	Examples
'Buddy' or mentor	Clinical placement facility	Role modelling Support Supervision of clinical practice related to patient care Contribute to assessment by feedback to student and faculty staff/clinical teacher	An RN in the acute psychiatric unit at a public hospital works with the second-year student for three shifts during the 2-week placement. Together they care for the four patients allocated to the RN, with the student assuming full responsibility (within her scope of practice) for the care of two of the patients. The RN provides feedback about the student's performance to the student and the clinical teacher each shift.
Preceptor	Clinical placement facility	Role modelling Support Supervision of clinical practice related to patient care Assessment of competence (often in consultation with faculty staff/clinical teacher)	An RN on the orthopaedic ward at a private hospital is the third-year student's preceptor over a 4-week period. The student gradually assumes full responsibility (within his scope of practice) for the four patients allocated to the preceptor. He discusses his care planning with his preceptor and asks her if he is unsure, but otherwise he works as independently as possible. A lecturer from the university visits the student and preceptor three times each week. They both provide performance feedback to the student and set clinical learning activities. The preceptor completes the student's competency assessment in consultation with the faculty lecturer.
Clinical educator/clinical facilitator/clinical teacher/clinical supervisor	Educational institution (faculty) (e.g. a lecturer or a sessional clinical teacher *or* an RN—could be a clinician or nurse educator—who normally works at the facility who is seconded for the duration of the placement to work for the faculty)	Clinical teaching Role modelling Support Supervision of clinical skills (as arranged with facility) Assessment of competence	The clinical teacher has a group of eight first-year students who are completing a 2-week clinical placement at a nursing home. Each student is 'buddied' with a nurse from the nursing home, and performs care for the residents within their scope of practice. During the shift, the clinical teacher spends time with each student. She assists in direct care (e.g. hygiene), demonstrates clinical skills (e.g. documentation) and arranges for the group to attend the weekly in-service education sessions (e.g. about managing incontinence). At the end of each shift, she conducts a 30-minute debriefing and education session where the students discuss their experiences and review topics of interest. The clinical teacher provides feedback to the students about their performance each shift, sets learning activities and completes formal assessments for each student.

Educational institution requirements and expectations

Make sure that you attend all clinical placement briefing sessions conducted at your educational institution. Before starting the placement, you should read the faculty clinical education policy. You will need to know the location of the facility, and the ward, unit or area where you are allocated, the duration and roster for your clinical placement. You will also need to know the uniform requirements, meeting place for the first day, and the name and contact details of your clinical teacher, mentor, preceptor or faculty contact. You will be expected to wear your student identification badge during the clinical placement. Most educational institutions will remind its students that they represent the institution and are visitors in the clinical placement facility. You will be expected to behave accordingly.

Clinical teacher's requirements and expectations

Your clinical teacher will have specific expectations, which are directly related to your clinical placement. Your clinical teacher is employed—or contracted—by your educational institution and will be familiar with the curriculum and the broad objectives for the clinical placement. The clinical teacher will provide you with details for contacting him or her during the placement, and will advise you of how the supervision, teaching and assessment will occur.

For example, the clinical teacher might attend handover with each student over the course of the placement, arrange times to observe you working or performing specific skills, such as drug administration, negotiate a time each shift for you to handover your patients, and advise you when and how the interim and final assessments will take place. Your clinical teacher will expect you to discuss your learning objectives each shift, and to be able to discuss the care of the patients allocated to you. The clinical teacher will also set key learning activities, such as developing a nursing care plan, completing a drug diary or presenting a handover to the group. If you are unsure of your clinical teacher's expectations, it is important that you ask.

Clinical placement facility requirements and expectations

The clinical placement facility will have certain requirements and expectations of you. You should research the facility, including its history, mission and the type of services it offers before starting your placement. As a visitor in the facility, you will be expected to be courteous and respectful. While you are at the facility, you represent both the facility and your educational institution. You must wear your student identification, the appropriate uniform and take any equipment you need (e.g. pens, watch with a second hand). You will need to be punctual and arrive prepared for your shift.

You should be orientated to the physical environment and specific policies, procedures or practices of the facility and the particular ward, unit or area where you are allocated. Always ensure that you know the emergency codes and the location of emergency equipment. (Orientation is discussed in detail in Ch 13.) You might need to observe particular requests about car parking, use of staff facilities or security.

Learning requirements and expectations

Your educational institution and the clinical placement facility will both expect that you are aware of the type of experience you will have (e.g. acute adult care in a public hospital) and the **learning objectives** you need to achieve.

While your educational institution will have specified some of the expected learning outcomes related to the clinical placement, along with the method of assessment and the competencies you will be expected to demonstrate, it is important for you to reflect on your expectations—of the clinical placement, of the educational institution, of your clinical teacher and of yourself.

QUESTION FOR REFLECTION

What are your expectations of clinical placement?

You will also be expected to develop your own learning objectives and identify your learning needs. This will include stating your strengths and identifying areas for development. When writing your own leaning objectives before the clinical placement, you should list specific strategies for achieving your goals (see Table 12.2). Remember also that the achievement of certain competencies could be the basis of a learning objective. Use the 'Learning objectives template' (R6.2), in the 'Clinical placement folio' on the CD Part 3—Reader resources, for writing your own objectives.

TABLE 12.2 Sample learning objectives

Area for development	Goal	Strategies
Drug calculations	To be competent in all drug calculations	Complete drug calculations worksheet before clinical placement Attend drug calculations tutorial before clinical placement Check all drug calculations with RN on clinical placement Ask clinical teacher to test me on drug calculations during placement
Handover	To be confident and competent at handover	Listen to the CD Part 1—Audio, 'Nursing handovers' (A15–A16) Use the hospital handover sheet Write handover notes Practise handover with clinical teacher before giving handover to staff

In addition, you should be familiar with the relevant **competency standards** (as discussed in Ch 5) and the **competency assessment tool** used by your educational institution (see Ch 13). It is essential to have a very clear understanding of the competencies you must demonstrate in order to successfully complete the clinical placement. (See Ch 13 for a discussion of competency assessment.)

QUESTION FOR REFLECTION

What are your strengths and areas for development?

CHAPTER HIGHLIGHTS

- Clinical placements are an essential component of most nursing courses in Australia and New Zealand, as specified by the nursing regulatory authorities.
- Clinical placements provide opportunities for praxis and reflection.
- Clinical placements occur in a variety of settings.
- Clinical education and support is provided to nursing students by various models of clinical supervision.
- Educational institutions and clinical placement agencies have requirements and expectations of nursing students.
- Nursing students are expected to be cognisant of the key learning outcomes for the placement, the method of assessment and the competencies to be met.
- Nursing students are expected to reflect on their expectations and learning needs.
- Essential preparation for clinical placement includes the development of learning objectives, the revision of competency standards, a review of the (educational institution's) specific competency assessment tool, and a clear understanding of the competency requirements for the placement.

Self-test questions

1. Describe the purpose of clinical placements.
2. Provide definitions of praxis and reflection.
3. Why is the educational institution responsible for the employment of clinical teachers?
4. Using examples, differentiate between a mentor, a preceptor and a clinical teacher.
5. List the general expectations an educational institution and a clinical placement facility could have of nursing students.
6. Review your educational institution's policies and regulations regarding clinical placements.
7. Review the (national) competency standards for nurses, which are most relevant to you.
8. Review your educational institution's clinical placement competency assessment tool.
9. After reflecting on your current level of experience with clinical placements, develop a set of learning objectives using the 'Learning objectives template' (R6.2), in the 'Clinical placement folio' (R6) on the CD Part 3—Reader resources.
10. Read and summarise a recent local journal article about clinical placements using the 'Article summary sheet' (R1) on the CD Part 3—Reader resources.
11. Review the key terms and any other new vocabulary, terms and abbreviations from this chapter, and then update your 'Language list' (R2) on the CD Part 3—Reader resources.
12. Answer the 'Learning objectives' at the start of this chapter as if they were examination questions.

References

Alliex S, McCarthy A 2005 Reflective practice: retrospective reality and rhetoric or strategies to enhance clinical practice? In: The reflective practitioner. Proceedings of the 14th Annual Teaching Learning Forum, 3–4 February 2005, Murdoch University, Perth. Online. Available http://lsn.curtin.edu.au/tlf/tlf2005/refereed/alliex.html 24 Dec 2007

Australian Nursing and Midwifery Council 2002 National Competency Standards for the Enrolled Nurse. Online. Available www.anmc.org.au/docs/Publications/Competency%20 standards%20EN.pdf 23 Oct 2007

Australian Nursing and Midwifery Council 2006 National Competency Standards for the Registered Nurse. Online. Available www.anmc.org.au/docs/Competency_standards_ RN.pdf 23 Oct 2007

Bulman C 2004 An introduction to reflection. In Bulman C, Schutz S (eds) Reflective practice in nursing, 3rd edn. Blackwell, Oxford, pp 1–24

Levett-Jones T, Bourgeois S 2007 The clinical placement: an essential guide for nursing students. Elsevier, Sydney

Mills JE, Francis KL, Bonner A 2005 Mentoring, clinical supervision and preceptoring: clarifying the conceptual definitions for Australian rural nurses. A review of the literature. Rural and Remote Health 5 (online) 2005: 410. Online. Available www.rrh.org.au/articles/ subviewnew.asp?ArticleID=410 20 Dec 2007

Nursing Council of New Zealand 2007a Competencies for nurse assistants and enrolled nurses. Online. Available www.nursingcouncil.org.nz/NA%20Comps%20final.pdf 14 May 2008

Nursing Council of New Zealand 2007b Competencies for registered nurses. Online. Available www.nursingcouncil.org.nz/RN%20Comps%20final.pdf 14 May 2008

Rolfe G 1993 Closing the theory–practice gap: a model of nursing praxis. Journal of Clinical Nursing 2(3):173–177

Rolfe G 2006 Nursing praxis and the science of the unique. Nursing Science Quarterly 19:39–43

Tarlier D 2005 Mediating the meaning of evidence through epidemiological diversity. Nursing Inquiry 12(2):126–134

Recommended reading

Levett-Jones T, Bourgeois S 2007 The clinical placement: an essential guide for nursing students. Elsevier, Sydney

CHAPTER 13

During clinical placement . . .

'I want to be a very safe nurse and show that I am a competent nurse, so then I will be able to get a job here. This is my dream . . . and clinical experience is a very important way to show I can be a nurse here in the future.'

Park, South Korea

CHAPTER OUTLINE

LEARNING OBJECTIVES

1. Discuss in detail the expectations of nursing students during clinical placements.
2. Provide specific examples of safe, legal and ethical practice for student nurses.
3. Discuss the concepts of accountability and responsibility in nursing.
4. Describe theory, practice and praxis in nursing.
5. Discuss in detail the student nurse's responsibilities when performing clinical skills during clinical placements.
6. Become familiar with the types of clinical skills performed by nurses in Australia and New Zealand.
7. Identify the key clinical skills for international nurses.
8. Describe and utilise the nursing process for patient care.
9. Describe strategies for effective time management during the clinical placement.
10. Describe the process of competency assessment in the clinical placement.
11. Develop a personal plan for learning during clinical placements.
12. Develop a personal plan for demonstrating competence during clinical placements.

Key terms (are in bold in the text)

accountability
ADPIE
assessment
assessor
clinical educator
clinical experience
clinical facility
clinical placements
clinical skills
clinical supervisor
clinical teacher
competency assessment tool
competency standards
contextual knowledge
countersign
diagnosis
educational institution
emergency codes
evaluation
implementation
interventions
learning objectives
nursing diagnosis
nursing process
patient allocation
planning
praxis
prioritising
psychomotor skills
reflection
reflective practice
responsibility
scope of practice
self-assessment
supernumerary
theoretical knowledge
time management

Clinical placements can provide some of the most exciting, rewarding and challenging experiences for nursing students. Being well prepared and maximising the learning opportunities available will help to ensure your success in developing and demonstrating competence during the clinical placement.

If you are an overseas registered nurse—but are not registered in Australia or New Zealand—remember that during clinical placements you will be considered a student nurse. While it can be difficult to be a student again, it is important to use the opportunities available during clinical placements to experience nursing in another culture and context, to reflect on the similarities and differences between nursing in your country, to learn new clinical skills and to develop your communication skills.

It is strongly recommended that you read a text that addresses clinical placement issues, listed in the 'Recommended reading' (Levett-Jones & Bourgeois 2007).

The student nurse on clinical placement

There are a number of expectations of nursing students—and overseas nurses completing pre-registration supervised practice—during **clinical placements**. Some of these reflect the need for professional behaviour, some are to ensure safe, legal and ethical practice, and others relate to how students can meet **learning objectives**. It is likely that your **educational institution** will brief you about the following expectations and your responsibilities before the clinical placement commences.

Arrival

It is important to arrive a little early at the **clinical facility** on your first day of clinical placement. You will be expected to meet your **clinical teacher**, also sometimes called **clinical educator** or **clinical supervisor**, at a designated place (e.g. the hospital reception) or to go directly to the ward/unit/area and locate the nominated contact person (e.g. to meet the nurse unit manager (NUM) in the conference room at the nursing home). Punctuality for all shifts and scheduled activities is expected.

Presentation

You will need to wear appropriate attire (often this will be the educational institution's uniform, which should be correct, clean and ironed) and abide by the facility's uniform policy. Many places will restrict the type of jewellery that can be worn, require long hair to be tied back, fingernails to be short and unvarnished, and state that flat, closed shoes must be worn in clinical areas. For security and identification, you should wear your student identification badge and it should be clearly visible at all times.

Introductions

At times, you will need to introduce yourself to facility staff. Always be clear that you are a student nurse (so that people do not assume you are a registered nurse or a permanent member of staff). You could say: 'My name is Sue Ibraham and I am a second-year nursing student from Happy Valley university. I am doing my community nursing placement here. I'll be here for 2 weeks'. You never need to apologise for being a student, so avoid saying, 'I am only a student' or 'I am just a student'.

Orientation

Orientation is a very important part of clinical placement, and will vary widely. As part of your preclinical placement preparation (outlined in Ch 12), you should have researched the facility. You should also be aware of the type of **clinical experience** you will have during the placement (e.g. acute paediatric).

To learn more about the 'typical' patient cases and the care provided in the specific ward/unit/area, you should research your medical–surgical nursing texts. If you have been allocated to the renal unit, it would be useful to read about renal conditions and the nursing care of people with renal conditions. At the start of the placement, you will learn the common admission diagnoses of patients in the unit, and can complete further research then.

On the first day of the clinical placement, ensure that you are orientated. If there is not a formal orientation program, it is your responsibility to ask the staff or your clinical teacher what you need to know. You need to know the location of the ward/unit/area in the facility, the entrances and exits, lifts and stairs, and the physical layout of the ward/unit/area, as well as the location of staff facilities (such as the tea room, cafeteria and toilets). It is essential to know the emergency codes and procedures, and the location and use of emergency equipment, the patient call bell system and telephones. Find out the location of important items and equipment, such as sterile supplies, patient files and medications, at the start of the placement. Use the 'Orientation checklist' (R6.3), in the 'Clinical placement folio' (R6) on the CD Part 3—Reader resources, to assist you.

Ensure that you know where to meet on the second day of placement (e.g. the handover room at the start of the shift), and also where to meet your clinical teacher for debriefing if you are required to attend.

Supervision and education

Suitable registered nurses must supervise nursing students at all times during clinical placements. As the educational institution is ultimately responsible for the clinical education of its students (as discussed in Ch 12), it has an important role in ensuring that appropriate supervision of nursing students occurs.

The nursing regulatory authorities also stipulate that nursing students must be **supernumerary**. This means that your presence is *in addition* to, not instead of, the usual nursing staff numbers. As you are not replacing a nurse, you can feel confident using the clinical experience as an opportunity to learn, not simply to work.

Irrespective of the model of supervision, education and support used during your clinical placement, you should be clear about which registered nurse is responsible for working with you. You must know to whom you should report information about the patients you have been allocated (remember a registered nurse is still responsible for supervising you and for the care of those patients) and who to ask to explain something you do not understand. If you are uncertain and you have a clinical teacher, you should always feel free to ask your clinical teacher.

If you experience any difficulties with the supervision of your clinical placement, you should contact the clinical teacher or, if you are experiencing a problem with the clinical teacher, the appropriate person at your educational institution immediately. Ensure that you have appropriate evidence of the problem, and report it objectively.

Patient allocation

It is important for nursing students to have the experience of assuming responsibility and accountability for the care of patients—within their **scope of practice** and limitations as a student nurse. This is widely recognised in nursing education and practice, and in many clinical placements **patient allocation** will occur. This means that you will be allocated patients based on your experience and competence. You should also always know which registered nurse is responsible for supervising you and ultimately for the care of 'your' patients. You must also know about the condition and care for each of your patients (as outlined in Table 13.2).

Absenteeism

If you will be absent from the placement or you are running late for your shift, you must contact the appropriate person (e.g. your clinical teacher, a faculty member, your preceptor or the NUM). Ensure you obtain the details of the person to whom you reported your absenteeism, particularly if they are going to convey the message.

Managing unexpected events

At times, nursing students must manage unexpected events. If you are involved in a situation that requires the use of an incident report (see Ch 11), such as a drug administration error, a needlestick injury, or you witness a patient fall, you must complete the facility incident report, and, if required, provide a copy for your educational institution or complete a separate incident report. You must notify the registered nurse who is supervising you immediately, and notify your clinical teacher or a faculty member as soon as possible after the incident. If you have a clinical teacher, he or she will usually assist you to write the incident report (and check your draft documentation). If you do not have a clinical teacher, ask the registered nurse supervising you to assist.

During clinical placements, students can be involved in emergency situations. All facilities have **emergency codes** (e.g. Code Blue for cardiac arrest), but these are not universal, so you must be familiar with the codes, policies and procedures for managing emergencies in every clinical placement facility you attend. You will need to know what telephone numbers to dial, what to say and what is expected of the staff in an emergency. Remember that even in an emergency, nursing students must practise within their scope of practice and limitations, although you will be expected to be able to call a code and locate and deliver the emergency equipment to the scene. (See Table13.1 for an example of student nurse actions in a cardiac arrest.)

Student nurses are expected to be able to perform basic life support (BLS) before attending clinical placements, and to update this skill regularly. You should also know how to operate the patient call bell, and be able to use the features on the bed, including removing the head of the bed, changing the bed height, and operating cot sides/bed rails, steering controls and the brakes. (See the 'Orientation checklist' (R6.3) in the 'Clinical placement folio' (R6) on the CD Part 3—Reader resources.)

Not all unexpected events lead to medical emergencies. However, any unusual or abnormal findings, observations or assessments (e.g. the patient reports chest pain or the patient's pulse is tachycardic and irregular) must be reported to a registered nurse immediately.

A combination of knowledge, clinical skills and communication skills is essential for managing unexpected events during clinical placements.

Leaving the ward

Apart from being courteous, it is important for continuity of care and patient safety and security that you advise an appropriate person when leaving the ward/unit/area.

If you are leaving the clinical area during your shift (e.g. for a meeting with your clinical teacher, or for a meal break), you must tell the registered nurse supervising you, provide a handover and ask him or her to assume responsibility for your patients in your absence. You could say: 'Kerry, I am going to be with my clinical teacher in the conference room for about 15 minutes. Would you mind looking after Mr Saunders while I am gone? He returned to the ward after an appendicectomy at 1100 hr. His post-op

TABLE 13.1 Student nurse actions in a medical emergency

Instruction	Specific action	Example: student Sara Chan
Call a code	Dial emergency number (for facility) State code name State location State specific site	Dials 71 Says: 'Code Blue, ward 14, bed 7'
Bring emergency equipment to scene	Locate resuscitation trolley outside nurses' station Scene of emergency is bed 7	Goes to resuscitation trolley and takes resuscitation trolley to bed 7
Meet resuscitation team	Await team at lift 2	Meets resuscitation team at lift 2
Escort resuscitation team to patient	Lead team to scene	Says: 'Follow me to bed 7' Leads team to patient

vital signs are due in half an hour. They have been within normal limits. His dressing is dry and intact. His IV is running at 125 mL/hr via a pump and is on time. He had some pethidine at 1200 hr and says he is comfortable now. Thank you.'

When you finish your shift, say goodbye to the patients for whom you have been caring and tell them who is taking over their care (see the examples in Table 10.3 in the section on concluding conversations). Always ensure that the registered nurse supervising you knows when you leave the ward, and if it is not at the end of his or her shift, explain why you are leaving early and provide a handover. You could say: 'Thanks for working with me today, Max. It's 3 o'clock and we have a debrief with our clinical teacher now, until 3.30. I will be back tomorrow morning. I have done everything on my timeline. You have countersigned my notes, and Mrs Soo is having her chest X-ray. She has been gone about 10 minutes.'

You should not return to the clinical area after you have finished your shift—and certainly must *not* engage in any patient care. This is important because you must be supervised at all times by a registered nurse, and also because the educational institution and the clinical facility have contractual arrangements that specify when students are authorised to be in the facility.

QUESTION FOR REFLECTION

Are the expectations and responsibilities of nursing students different in your country?

QUESTION FOR REFLECTION

If you are an overseas nurse, how do you feel about being a 'student' nurse in Australia or New Zealand? How could this impact on your clinical placement?

Caring for patients

Providing care for 'real' patients during clinical placements is often a highlight of the clinical experience for nursing students. As the nursing student who is accountable and responsible for the care of the patient, you will be expected to have an extensive knowledge of the patient, to meet the patient's needs—within your scope of practice—to communicate using advanced verbal skills and documentation, and to manage your time during the shift. (See the ◉ 'Preparation for patient care document' (R6.6) in the 'Clinical placement folio' (R6) on the CD Part 3—Reader resources.)

Responsibility and accountability

It is essential for all nurses and nursing students to understand that they are responsible and accountable for their actions, and for the care of the patients whom they have been allocated. The legislation governing nursing and the professional codes, standards and competencies relevant to nursing in Australia and New Zealand all address these concepts (Australian Nursing and Midwifery Council 2002a, 2002b, 2003, 2006, New Zealand Ministry of Health 2006, Nursing Council of New Zealand 2007a, 2007b, 2008). (See Ch 5 for a detailed discussion of nursing standards and competencies.)

Remember that at all times you are responsible for practising within the limits of your knowledge and experience—that is, within the scope of your practice as a student nurse.

Knowing and doing

Having a sound knowledge base is an essential competency for nursing practice (Australian Nursing and Midwifery Council 2002b, 2006, Nursing Council of New Zealand 2007a, 2007b).

Knowledge is not limited to theory, but includes practical knowledge and the application of theory to practice. **Praxis** (as discussed in Ch 12) is an important concept in clinical education. The knowledge required for specific clinical skills is discussed below.

During clinical placement, students often ask, 'What do I need to know?' The answer is you need to know everything! That is, you need to know everything about your patient and about your nursing care, as outlined in Table 13.2. To develop your knowledge of patients' problems and nursing care, consult the texts listed in the 'Recommended reading' (Brown & Edwards 2008, Crisp & Taylor 2009, Elder et al 2008, Fortinash & Holoday Worret 2007).

In addition, you must be able to demonstrate competent nursing care of your patient, be able to document appropriately and 'hand over' the patient. (See the ◉ 'Preparation for patient care document' (R6.6) in the 'Clinical placement folio' (R6) on the CD Part 3—Reader resources.)

? QUESTION FOR REFLECTION

Have you always known 'what you need to know about your patients'? How can you ensure you have a safe knowledge base for practice?

Clinical skills

'Doing clinical skills' is one of the greatest areas of concern for nursing students, and there are a number of issues that must be understood. If you practise beyond your limitations and scope of practice (as a student nurse), or are involved in unsafe practice or practice that breaches laws or professional codes, policies, standards or competencies, you could fail your clinical placement.

TABLE 13.2 What you need to know about your patient

You need to know: • past medical history (and ongoing problems and care) • family history • allergies, sensitivities, intolerances (causal agents, reactions, usual management) • reason for admission • medical diagnosis • current or planned medical management • current nursing diagnoses • current or anticipated nursing care needs: all nursing care, clinical skills, medications, collaborative care • current condition and progress • special needs • referrals required • discharge planning

Clinical skills in your scope of practice

Nursing students are *not permitted* to perform clinical skills or to undertake activities for which they have not been prepared in their course of study. This includes the administration of medications and intravenous therapy. For example, if you have not learned about or practised a skill, such as removing a central venous catheter, it is *not* safe to perform this skill in the clinical setting. To do so would breach the competency standards that relate to patient safety, recognition of own scope of practice and limitations, accountability and responsibility, having an adequate knowledge base for safe practice and performing nursing interventions (Australian Nursing and Midwifery Council 2002b, 2006, Nursing Council of New Zealand 2007a, 2007b).

Supervision by a registered nurse

A registered nurse *must* supervise the performance of clinical skills by nursing students. The level of supervision varies according to the skill, the student's experience and the student's competence. For example, if you have learned about nasogastric intubation, have practised this in the clinical laboratories at your educational institution and, during the placement, you have an opportunity to perform the skill for the first time, this is an excellent learning opportunity. After revision and discussion of the skill parameters (in Table 13.3) with your clinical teacher or a registered nurse, you could perform the skill under the direct supervision of your clinical teacher or a registered nurse.

After you have demonstrated your competence in certain skills, such as assisting a patient with showering, or assessing vital signs, it is likely that you will be able to perform these skills without direct supervision. Always remember that you are responsible and accountable for your actions, and immediately report any unusual findings to a registered nurse.

You must be supervised when you are performing any skill for the first time, or when the skill is complex or invasive, involves medication or intravenous therapy administration, or if your clinical teacher or a registered nurse consider supervision to

TABLE 13.3 Parameters of clinical skill performance

Parameter	Example: nasogastric intubation
Theoretical knowledge (related to skill) *Knowing why*	Knows about the intervention: purpose, indications, contraindications, special care, potential complications Knows about the skill performance: procedure, rationales, management of complications
Psychomotor skills *Knowing how and doing*	Able to insert NGT competently
Contextual knowledge (related to the specific patient and the skill) *Knowing and doing = praxis*	Knows why Mrs Tan has NGT (i.e. for decompression of gastric contents, not for enteral feeding, so the NGT is connected to a drainage bag and 4-hourly aspiration of the tube is planned, and a FBC is commenced)

be appropriate. You should ask to be supervised if you have any concerns. Even after registration, it is appropriate to observe another nurse perform a new or complex skill before attempting it, and to ask to be supervised when performing any skill for the first time.

Abiding by the law

Students are *not permitted* to perform any skill or activity that the law—or facility policy—requires is performed only by a registered nurse. It is a competency requirement that nursing practice is legal and upholds local policies (Australian Nursing and Midwifery Council 2002b, 2006, Nursing Council of New Zealand 2007a, 2007b). For example, the administration of drugs is restricted to certain health professionals, by law. Student nurses must not administer medication without being directly supervised by a registered nurse, who must **countersign** the drug chart, after the drug is administered (this means the student and the registered nurse both sign). If the facility policy requires two registered nurses to check the injectable drugs before administration, then two registered nurses must check—and the student can also check, in addition to the two registered nurses, but not instead of one of the registered nurses.

Performance versus competence

Clinical skill performance is *not the same as* being competent at the clinical skill. Remember that simply 'doing' a skill—without adequate knowledge—is potentially very unsafe and breaches nursing competency standards (Australian Nursing and Midwifery Council 2002b, 2006, Nursing Council of New Zealand 2007a, 2007b). To be considered competent at a skill, you must be competent in all the parameters of skill performance outlined in Table 13.3.

Medication and intravenous therapy administration are clinical skills that will be assessed according to the parameters of clinical skill performance (in Table 13.3). For example, if a student gave an IM injection of morphine to a patient, and was able to demonstrate her **theoretical knowledge**, including a sound knowledge of morphine, and **psychomotor skills**, but she did not know why that patient had been prescribed morphine (i.e. she lacked the **contextual knowledge** required), she would be deemed unsafe and fail to meet the competency standards related to safety, accountability and responsibility, having an adequate knowledge base for safe practice and performing nursing interventions (Australian Nursing and Midwifery Council 2002b, 2006, Nursing Council of New Zealand 2007a, 2007b).

Clinical skills performance is not the same as overall competence in clinical practice. Many students worry that they have limited opportunities to become proficient in 'skills' and during clinical placements are keen to do as many skills as possible, as often as possible. It is very important to remember that nursing practice is not limited to clinical skills, and that to be competent you must meet nursing competency standards—and not simply tick off a list of skills!

There will be some clinical skills that you will not have the opportunity to perform as a nursing student. As a registered nurse, you are responsible for ensuring that you are supervised when performing a new or complex skill for the first time.

?

QUESTION FOR REFLECTION

Before reading this chapter, how would you have measured clinical skill competence?

Additional clinical skills

The additional key clinical skills for overseas nurses and international nursing students are listed in Table 13.4. It is very important to allow time to become proficient in those clinical skills that depend on communication. Remember that it is a nursing competency requirement that you *can communicate effectively in English* (Australian Nursing and Midwifery Council 2002b, 2006, Nursing Council of New Zealand 2007a, 2007b). Apart from their importance for safe practice, communication skills are essential for you to demonstrate your competence. To develop your communication skills, review Chapters 2, 10 and 11. Listen to the CD Part 1—Audio, complete the activities and self-test questions in Part 7 of the text, and complete the self-directed learning packages on the CD Part 3—Reader resources.

TABLE 13.4 Additional key clinical skills for international nurses

Verbal communication (see Chs 2, 7, 8, 9 and 10)
• nursing admission interview
• instructing patients about mobilising and positioning
• handover
Documentation (see Ch 11)
• nursing charts (as listed in Table 11.1)
• nursing care plans
• clinical/critical pathways
• progress notes
• referral letters
Clinical skills
• refer to a clinical skills text
• drug diary
• refer to a nursing calculations text

To develop your knowledge of medications, use a drug diary. (See the 'Drug diary' (R6.9) in the 'Clinical placement folio' (R6) on the CD Part 3—Reader resources.) To practise drug and intravenous therapy calculations, consult the nursing calculations text listed in the 'Recommended reading' (Gatford & Phillips 2006). (See the 'Drug calculations and intravenous therapy formulas' (R6.10) in the 'Clinical placement folio' (R6) on the CD Part 3—Reader resources.)

To develop your psychomotor skills, consult a clinical skills text listed in the 'Recommended reading' (Perry & Potter 2005, Tollefson 2004). Always check the facility policy regarding clinical skills. Some facilities require registered nurses to have specialised training before certain skills can be performed (e.g. IV cannulation), and there are some skills performed by registered nurses in Australia and New Zealand that are performed by medical staff in other countries (e.g. nasogastric intubation). (See the 'Preparation for clinical skills checklist' (R6.7) in the 'Clinical placement folio' (R6) on the CD Part 3—Reader resources.)

?

QUESTION FOR REFLECTION

Reflect on your current experience, and consider how confident you feel about your competence in each of the clinical skills listed in Table13.4. How will you develop your competence?

The nursing process

The **nursing process** is 'a series of steps that provides a framework for addressing problems' (Fitzgerald 2008 p 15). While it has been widely critiqued (Varcoe 1996), the nursing process does provide a model for considering how nurses assess, plan and deliver care.

The nursing process is a critical thinking competency in nursing (Jones 2009 Ch 14). The ability to use the nursing process is a nursing competency requirement in Australia and New Zealand (Australian Nursing and Midwifery Council 2002b, 2006, Nursing Council of New Zealand 2007a, 2007b).

The phases of the nursing process can be remembered by the acronym **ADPIE** (this is similar to the formats for narrative style documentation discussed in Ch 11). While the process is represented as sequential phases, assessment and evaluation occur throughout, and a nurse can move between phases, depending on the data available as the nurse cares for the patient (Fitzgerald 2008 p 18). Figure 13.1 describes the key phases of the nursing process.

The nursing process can be used in documentation, and is incorporated into problem-based nursing care plans and problem-based progress notes, which reflect phases of the nursing process (as discussed in Ch 11). It is also possible to use the nursing process in a problem-based handover (see Table 10.4).

Time management

Time management is an essential skill for nurses, and this is reflected in the nursing competency standards (Australian Nursing and Midwifery Council 2002b, 2006, Nursing Council of New Zealand 2007a, 2007b). The elements of time management include the ability to prioritise care, to adapt to changing situations and emergencies, and to provide care in an efficient and timely manner.

Time management develops with experience and confidence. During clinical placements, students' time management skills can be improved using a number of key strategies. The use of timelines is recommended. (See the 'Timeline template' (R6.5) in the 'Clinical placement folio' (R6) on the CD Part 3—Reader resources.) Remember

FIGURE 13.1 The nursing process

A—Assessment (admission interview, history and physical examination, data collection)

Assessment involves obtaining assessment data from the patient and, where appropriate, from other relevant sources (including family members, and the patient's file or medical records, emergency service admission form or referral letters).

It includes subjective and objective data, and the clinical manifestations (signs and symptoms) with which a patient presents.

↓

D—Diagnosis (nursing diagnosis, patient problems)

Problem framing is required in this phase. Using the assessment data, the nurse develops a set of 'problems' that the patient is experiencing (actual) or might experience (potential).

The nursing diagnosis is not the medical diagnosis (of an illness or condition).

When the nursing and medical problems are considered jointly, they are referred to as collaborative problems.

The diagnoses must be patient/client focused.

↓

P—Planning (or **prioritising**, goal setting, care planning)

The planning phase involves a number of steps:

- determining priorities
- setting goals
- determining appropriate care (based on the nursing diagnosis)
- planning evaluation of the interventions, along with reassessment of the patient.

The planning must be patient/client focused.

↓

I—Implementation (or **interventions**, nursing care, care, treatment)

During this phase, the nurse implements the care to address the diagnosis and to achieve the goal. The nurse must be able to provide rationales for care.

Some interventions are medical initiatives, and are sometimes referred to as collaborative interventions.

↓

E—Evaluation (or review, audit, reassessment)

During this phase, the nurse evaluates the interventions, based on goals. Interventions should address the problem. Modification of the diagnosis, the plan and interventions should occur where required.

Assessment occurs again after evaluation.

also to ask your clinical teacher, preceptor or mentor for assistance to develop your time management skills. For example, discuss your timeline with your mentor at the start of the shift. This helps you to clarify the way you have prioritised your care, provides an opportunity for your mentor to remind you of anything you have omitted, and allows you to benefit from the role modelling or suggestions your mentor makes.

It is also important to be as prepared as possible for the shift. For example, if you know in advance which patients you will be allocated, research their conditions and medications, and practise the clinical skills you will need to perform. The more confident you feel about your knowledge and skills, the more time efficient you will be. Ensure you are up to date with the theoretical and practical knowledge you are expected to have!

Reflection

As discussed in Chapter 12, clinical placement also provides the opportunity for **reflection** or **reflective practice** (Levett-Jones & Bourgeois 2007 pp 116–21). It is expected that you will be able to demonstrate your ability to reflect on your practice, as it is a specific competency requirement for nurses in Australia and New Zealand (Australian Nursing and Midwifery Council 2002b, 2006, Nursing Council of New Zealand 2007a, 2007b). Often, students are asked to keep a journal, in which they record their experiences, including their actions, thoughts and feelings, during clinical placement. Reflecting on your clinical performance can assist you in self-assessment of your competency.

Assessment of competency during clinical placement

Most clinical placement assessments are competency-based, and the majority of tools reflect standard competencies. As advised in Chapter 12, you will need to be familiar with the **competency standards** (as discussed in Ch 5), the **competency assessment tool** used by your educational institution, and how **assessors** determine competence.

Competency assessment tools

The competency assessment tool will have the key features outlined in Table 13.5.

Assessing competence

During the clinical placement, the person responsible for assessing your competence will use a variety of methods to complete a 'global assessment of [your] knowledge, skills, attitudes, values and abilities' (Australian Nursing and Midwifery Council 2002c p 8). To be considered competent, you will need to demonstrate your competence in *all* of the required domains, units or elements. Your scope of practice and level of experience as a student or a nurse will be taken into consideration (see Table 13.5).

The methods used by an assessor could include observation, interviewing others (e.g. nurses, patients), auditing and analysis of documentation, testing and interviewing you and asking for your self-assessment (Australian Nursing and Midwifery Council 2002c pp 9–11). This data is measured against the competency standards to determine whether or not your clinical performance meets the standards.

TABLE 13.5 Competency assessment tools

Key feature	Example
Uses recognised and endorsed competency standards	The university in Australia uses a tool based on the ANMC National Competency Standards for the Registered Nurse. The university or polytechnic in New Zealand uses a tool based on the Nursing Council of New Zealand Competencies for the Registered Nurse.
Specifies the minimum competency level required	General competency is required in all domains (the assessor must take into account the scope of practice and experience of the student). *Or:* A scale is used and specifies the standard required (e.g. third-year Bachelor of Nursing students must demonstrate independent practice in all domains, while second-year Bachelor of Nursing students must demonstrate independent practice in Domain 1 and assisted practice in the other domains).
Has a legend or cues to describe the competency level required (where used)	A scale is used to define terms (e.g. independent practice is defined as requiring minimal guiding cues).

Remember that clinical skills are not the sole determinant of competence, and that in the assessment of clinical skills, theoretical knowledge, psychomotor skill and contextual knowledge are needed as evidence of competence in a clinical skill.

The Australian Nursing and Midwifery Council has developed principles to guide assessors in competency assessment (2002c), and these are listed in Table 13.6. It is useful for students to also be aware of these principles. Although not formally adopted by the Nursing Council of New Zealand, these principles are equally applicable for New Zealand nurses—and students.

?

QUESTION FOR REFLECTION

Have you previously considered how competence is assessed? How does your developing awareness of the competency assessment process change your approach to clinical placements?

Meeting competency standards

It is often helpful to remember that to find that you are competent—for your scope of practice and level of experience—the assessor will assess your clinical performance and must provide evidence of your competence. This is also true when determining that a person has not met the competency standard required. Table 13.7 describes strategies you can implement to demonstrate your level of competence. The rationales reflect the relevant parameters of competence (skills, knowledge, attitudes, values and abilities).

?

QUESTION FOR REFLECTION

Reflect on how you have used—or could use—the strategies in Table 13.7. Which ones are difficult for you and how can you develop confidence in using them?

TABLE 13.6 Principles for assessing competence

Principle	Implications
1. Accountability	The assessor is accountable to the profession, the organisation (i.e. the faculty, nursing regulatory authority), and the person being assessed.
2. Performance-based assessment	Assessment must be based on clinical performance—in a clinical setting—over time.
3. Contextual relevance	The competence must be relevant in the clinical setting.
4. Evidence-based assessment	The assessor must provide evidence to support the assessment finding.
5. Validity and reliability in assessment	The process must be valid (test is appropriate) and reliable (consistent). The assessor's knowledge and skills are critical.
6. Participation and collaboration	The relationship between the assessor and person being assessed is important. Communication, impartiality and reflection are essential.

Source: Australian Nursing and Midwifery Council 2002c pp 12–15.

TABLE 13.7 Strategies to demonstrate competence

Strategy	Rationale	Examples
Be prepared for the placement and for every shift	Reflects positive attitude and values	Research the facility and the common conditions of patients in the unit. Arrive punctually, have a handover sheet, have all personal items required (e.g. watch, pens, ID). You *must* be familiar with the competency standards and the tool being used.
Ask questions—to learn more, for clarification or if unsure (especially about scope of practice issues)	Reflects positive attitude and values; allows demonstration of knowledge and abilities. Use of communication is critical to the demonstration of competence.	Ask: 'Could you tell me more about that procedure? I will also research it tonight.' Say: 'Did you say NIDDM or IDDM? I did not quite hear you.' Ask [the clinical teacher]: 'My "buddy" said I could do Mr Jamil's dressing. I have not done a complex dressing before. Is this OK?'
Assume responsibility and accountability—for your learning, nursing care and actions	Reflects positive attitude and values; allows demonstration of knowledge, skills and abilities	Research anything of which you are unsure (e.g. patient's condition, drugs, a clinical skill). Read the patient file, recent progress notes and current charts at the start of the shift. Clarify any queries after handover. Know everything about your patients. Report all condition changes or patient problems.

(Continued)

TABLE 13.7 Strategies to demonstrate competence—*cont'd*

Strategy	Rationale	Examples
		Never exceed your scope of practice. Report errors or incidents immediately.
Be proactive—in seeking learning opportunities, in meeting your learning objectives, and in the assessment process	Reflects positive attitude and values; allows demonstration of knowledge, skills and abilities Demonstrates the ability to be a reflective practitioner Use of communication is critical to the demonstration of competence	Do not avoid opportunities (ask for support or assistance if you are anxious): Say: 'I would like to admit a patient today. I have not done this since last year. Could I go through the form with you first?' Say: 'We have learnt about and practised putting up IV fluids. Could I watch you the first time, and then would you supervise me the next time?' Meet your objectives: Say: 'I need practice with drug calculations. Could I do some with you later today?' Do not wait to be asked: Say [to assessor]: 'I have completed a nursing care plan and updated my drug diary. Could you please check them and give me some feedback?' Say [to clinical teacher]: 'Can I hand over my patients to you now?' Say [at start of shift to mentor]: 'I have done a timeline. Could you please check it.' Complete self-assessments. Ask for interim feedback.

'Failing' an assessment for a clinical placement is a very distressing event. For international students, it can also pose additional stress related to isolation from support networks, the financial burden of repeating subjects, the possibility of visas expiring before completing the course (if the course duration will be extended because of the failed placement) and, for some, the cultural issues associated with academic performance.

If you disagree with the assessment of your performance—and have carefully considered and reflected on the feedback provided—you can address your concerns through a grievance procedure. It is expected that all organisations that conduct competency assessments have a grievance procedure in place. See Table 13.8 for strategies to assist you if you have difficulty meeting the competency standard required during a clinical placement.

QUESTION FOR REFLECTION

Complete the following: 'If I failed a clinical placement, I would be most likely to . . .' Reflect on the strategies that can assist competence development, and focus on positive actions (not emotions).

TABLE 13.8 Strategies for dealing with 'failing' a clinical placement

Strategy	Further suggestions/rationales
Remain professional	Rude, aggressive behaviour is not acceptable. Assessment is a part of professional life.
Avoid blaming others	It is unprofessional to criticise the assessor or facility or others. The grievance procedure is the forum to objectively present your case.
Listen carefully to feedback	You will be advised of the domains/units/elements where you are not meeting/have not met the standard required. You will be given examples of why your performance did not meet the standard. (The assessor might provide an example and then discuss which competencies are involved, or review each competency in sequence and give examples.) You will be advised of specific strategies to improve your performance. During an interim (not final) assessment, you will be given timeframes for implementing the suggested strategies.
Ask questions	It is good to ask for more information, examples of your performance, clarification and, most importantly, for specific suggestions about how to improve.
Take notes	When upset, it can be difficult to recall what was said.
Complete a self-assessment (if you have not done so)	Allows time for reflection on your performance. Demonstrates to the assessor your understanding of the competency assessment process, competency standards and your belief about your performance. An honest self-assessment might be similar to the assessor's findings. Compare the self-assessment and assessor's assessment and discuss them.
Remember that: • not liking the finding is not the same as disagreeing with it • not liking a finding does not mean it is inaccurate • not agreeing with a finding does not mean it is not true (according to assessors)	Nobody expects a student to like 'failing' a clinical placement. It is a normal reaction to be upset and disappointed. You might agree with the finding. Try to see this as a learning opportunity, not as a personal failure. It is possible for the assessor and the student to have a different concept of competence. This will need to be resolved through acceptance and 'moving on' or via the grievance procedure.
Use the grievance procedure (of your educational institution)	You will need to ensure that you have grounds, or a legitimate reason, for appealing (see your institution's clinical education grievance policy and procedure). You must be objective and factual. You will be required to submit documentation and possibly appear before a panel to provide evidence of why your result should be altered. The outcomes could include: the result is not changed, you are given a chance to demonstrate your competence, or the result is changed (although there *must* be evidence of your competence for this to occur without reassessment).

(Continued)

TABLE 13.8 Strategies for dealing with 'failing' a clinical placement—*cont'd*

Strategy	Further suggestions/rationales
Accept the finding and 'move on'	If your appeal is unsuccessful, or you choose to accept the initial finding, it is important to have a plan for moving on. Firstly, remember that this is a learning opportunity. Remind yourself that 'failing' a placement does not mean you will fail other placements. Acknowledge that sometimes students need more time to meet the competencies. Focus on the competencies where you did not meet the standard, and write some learning objectives and specific strategies for meeting them (use the suggestions from your assessor). Take these objectives to the next (or repeated) clinical placement. If you feel comfortable and think it would assist you, it is acceptable to discuss the 'failed' placement with your next clinical teacher, preceptor or mentor—provided you focus on your learning needs (and avoid blaming others).

CHAPTER HIGHLIGHTS

- Nursing students are responsible for meeting key competencies related to professionalism, safety, legal and ethical practice during clinical placements.
- Patient allocation allows nursing students to experience essential aspects of nursing.
- Nurses and nursing students must assume responsibility and accountability for their actions, and for the care they provide.
- Knowledge, practice and praxis are critical concepts in clinical education.
- Nursing students are responsible for ensuring that they always practise within their limitations and their scope of practice as student nurses.
- Nursing students must be supervised during clinical placements. Clinical skills, including medication and intravenous therapy administration, must be directly supervised.
- Students must always meet legal requirements in their practice.
- Competence in clinical skills is determined by competence in theoretical and contextual knowledge, as well as psychomotor skills.
- The nursing process provides a framework for identifying and managing patient problems. The phases are: assessment; diagnosis; planning; implementation; and evaluation.
- Time management is an important skill for nursing students.
- Competency assessment focuses on global assessment of the key elements of competence—knowledge, skills, values, attitudes and abilities—in all of the competency domains/units/elements.
- Nursing students are advised to be prepared, ask questions, assume responsibility and accountability, and adopt a proactive approach to learning, demonstrating competence and assessment during clinical placements.

- If a student 'fails' a clinical placement, it is important to focus on the learning opportunity presented.

Self-test questions

1. Describe the expectations of nursing students during clinical placements. Provide examples of behaviours that meet professional, safety, legal and ethical competency standards.
2. Using clinical examples, discuss the concepts of accountability and responsibility as they relate to clinical placements for nursing students.
3. Using clinical examples, describe how theory, practice and praxis are related.
4. Discuss the student nurse's responsibilities when performing clinical skills during clinical placements.
5. List the parameters of clinical skill competence. Provide an example.
6. Explain why being able to perform a clinical skill is not the same as being competent at that clinical skill.
7. Identify the key clinical skills for international nurses and, after reflection on your current abilities, list some specific strategies to help you demonstrate competence in these skills.
8. Describe the nursing process.
9. Describe strategies for effective time management during the clinical placement.
10. Review your educational institution's policies and regulations regarding clinical placements, including the relevant grievance policy and procedures.
11. Review the (national) competency standards for nurses, which are most relevant to you.
12. Review your educational institution's clinical placement competency assessment tool.
13. Using examples, describe ways you can demonstrate your competence during clinical placement.
14. Explain why a student who manages his or her time well and completes many clinical skills efficiently, and is enthusiastic and confident, could be assessed as not meeting the competency standard required during his or her clinical placement.
15. Read and summarise a recent local journal article about competency assessment of clinical performance using the 'Article summary sheet' (R1) on the CD Part 3—Reader resources.
16. Review the documents in the 'Clinical placement folio' (R6) on the CD Part 3—Reader resources.
17. Review the key terms and any other new vocabulary, terms and abbreviations from this chapter, and then update your 'Language list' (R2) on the CD Part 3—Reader resources.
18. Answer the 'Learning objectives' at the start of this chapter as if they were examination questions.

References

Australian Nursing and Midwifery Council 2002a Code of Ethics for Nurses in Australia. Online. Available www.anmc.org.au/docs/ANMC_Code_of_Ethics.pdf 23 Oct 2007

Australian Nursing and Midwifery Council 2002b National Competency Standards for the Enrolled Nurse. Online. Available www.anmc.org.au/docs/Publications/Competency%20 standards%20EN.pdf 23 Oct 2007

Australian Nursing and Midwifery Council 2002c Principles for the assessment of National Competency Standards. Online. Available www.anmc.org.au/docs/Principles%20for%20the%20Assessment.pdf 23 Oct 2007
Australian Nursing and Midwifery Council 2003 Code of Professional Conduct for Nurses in Australia. Online. Available www.anmc.org.au/docs/ANMC_Professional_ Conduct.pdf 23 Oct 2007
Australian Nursing and Midwifery Council 2006 National Competency Standards for the Registered Nurse. Online. Available www.anmc.org.au/docs/Competency_standards_RN.pdf 23 Oct 2007
Fitzgerald M 2008 The importance of nursing. In: Brown D, Edwards H (eds) Lewis's medical–surgical nursing: assessment and management of clinical problems, 2nd edn. Elsevier, Sydney, pp 2–21
Jones B 2009 Critical thinking and nursing judgment. In: Crisp J, Taylor C (eds) Potter & Perry's fundamentals of nursing, 3rd edn. Elsevier, Sydney, Ch 14
Levett-Jones T, Bourgeois S 2007 The clinical placement: an essential guide for nursing students. Elsevier, Sydney
New Zealand Ministry of Health 2006 Health Practitioners Competence Assurance Act 2003. Online. Available www.moh.govt.nz/hpca 12 May 2007
Nursing Council of New Zealand 2007a Competencies for Nurse Assistants and Enrolled Nurses. Online. Available www.nursingcouncil.org.nz/NA%20Comps%20final.pdf 14 May 2008
Nursing Council of New Zealand 2007b Competencies for Registered Nurses. Online. Available www.nursingcouncil.org.nz/RN%20Comps%20final.pdf 14 May 2008
Nursing Council of New Zealand 2008 Code of Conduct for Nurses. Online. Available www.nursingcouncil.org.nz/code%20of%20conduct%20March%202008.pdf 14 May 2008
Varcoe C 1996 Disparagement of the nursing process: the new dogma? Journal of Advanced Nursing 23(1):120–125

Recommended reading

Brown D, Edwards H (eds) 2008 Lewis's medical–surgical nursing: assessment and management of clinical problems, 2nd edn. Elsevier, Sydney
Crisp J, Taylor C (eds) 2009 Potter & Perry's fundamentals of nursing, 3rd edn. Elsevier, Sydney
Elder R, Evans K, Nizette D (eds) 2008 Psychiatric and mental health nursing, 2nd edn. Elsevier, Sydney
Fortinash KM, Holoday Worret PA 2007 Psychiatric mental health nursing, 6th edn. Elsevier, Sydney
Gatford JD, Phillips N 2006 Nursing calculations, 7th edn. Elsevier, Sydney
Levett-Jones T, Bourgeois S 2007 The clinical placement: an essential guide for nursing students. Elsevier, Sydney
Perry AG, Potter PA 2005 Clinical nursing skills and techniques, 6th edn. Elsevier, St Louis
Tollefson J 2004 Clinical psychomotor skills: assessment tools for nursing students, 2nd edn. Social Science Press, Tuggerah

PART 6

Employment

CHAPTER 14

Preparing for employment[5]

'I have a job as PCA. I am learning more English because of my job. It will help me be confident to get a job here when I am a nurse.'

Na, Vietnam

CHAPTER OUTLINE

LEARNING OBJECTIVES

1. Become familiar with resources for finding employment as a nurse in Australia or New Zealand.
2. Prepare a curriculum vitae.
3. Develop confidence in writing job applications.
4. Identify the general requirements for job interviews.
5. Become familiar with the formats for job interviews.
6. Develop a personal plan for preparing for job interviews.

5 The author gratefully acknowledges the contribution of Julie Scott in advising about the general visa requirements for overseas workers.

Key terms (are in bold in the text)

- applicants
- applications
- application letter
- award
- curriculum vitae (CV)
- graduate program
- interview
- interviewers
- police check
- portfolio
- positions
- position description
- professional development
- referees
- references
- resumé
- wages

After you have met the conditions for registration as a nurse in Australia or New Zealand, and provided that you have an appropriate visa, you will be eligible to apply to work as a nurse. Some nursing students and overseas nurses also seek work as unregistered carers—personal care attendants (PCAs), personal carers or assistants in nursing (AINs) in Australia, or as healthcare assistants or personal care workers in New Zealand—while they are studying. This type of work can assist with understanding local healthcare systems and services, and also with English language development.

Applying for employment can be a very daunting experience and it is important that you have a clear understanding of the process involved. It is recommended that you access a booklet that advises student nurses about job applications, listed in the 'Recommended reading' (Queensland University of Technology 2005).

Applying for a job

Finding a job

Nursing **positions** are usually advertised in major newspapers and on the websites of employment agencies. If you are a student, ask your teachers the best local sources for job advertisements. It is possible that you will be eligible to apply for a **graduate program** at a hospital or other facility (but you will need to check with the facility, as graduate program positions are sometimes only available to permanent residents or citizens). If you have been completing a competency assessment program or supervised practice at an accredited facility (hospital), ask your program coordinator or a nurse educator about the best local sources for job advertisements, and if there is the possibility of employment at the facility after you are registered.

Positions and conditions

Advertisements for nursing positions will specify the level of nurse (e.g. RN), grade or experience ranking (e.g. RN Grade 2; RN level 2 or above), employment fraction (i.e. full time, part time or casual), tenure (e.g. permanent, 6-month contract), clinical area (e.g. medical ward, intensive care unit (ICU), thoracic surgery ward) and postgraduate qualifications (e.g. graduate certificate or higher degree in neonatal intensive care nursing). (See the 'Sample job advertisement' (R7.2) in the 'Job application folio' (R7) on the CD Part 3—Reader resources.)

Graduate nurse programs are offered in some hospitals and other facilities. These programs provide a range of clinical experiences for recent graduates, support through mentors, preceptors and clinical educators, as well as **professional development** and education opportunities. You must check your eligibility for a graduate program, and then apply as advised by the facility (either through a centralised application process or directly to the facility).

It is important to ensure that the employer is a legitimate organisation that provides working conditions and **wages** in accordance with the relevant **award** (employment agreement). The position advertisement will sometimes have a statement to this effect, and the **position description** certainly should. You should check the relevant nurses' awards with the nurses' unions in Australia (Australian Nursing Federation—ANF) or New Zealand (New Zealand Nurses Organisation—NZNO). (Contact details are in Ch 4.) Remember that nursing awards do not cover unregistered carers, but some nursing employment agencies do employ unregistered carers and can advise you further.

Job applications

Having decided that you meet the initial criteria for a position, you should follow the directions in the advertisement. You might be required to obtain a position description by telephoning, emailing or accessing the organisation's website. From the position description, you will develop an understanding of the type of clinical area, the roles and responsibilities related to the job, the organisation's management structure, the type of support available and the opportunities for professional development. (See the 'Sample position description' (R7.3) in the 'Job application folio' (R7) on the CD Part 3—Reader resources.) Carefully consider how your qualifications, skills, experience, interests and aspirations match the position and the organisation, and then decide whether or not to continue the application process.

Written **applications** are usually required for all positions. Typically, this includes submitting an application letter (or completing an application form from the employer) and a **curriculum vitae (CV)** or **resumé**. These provide the prospective employer with their first impression of you.

In Western culture, honesty is expected in job applications (similar to academic honesty as discussed in Ch 1), so ensure that your written application—and what you say at interview—is factual and accurate. Remember also that it is expected that nurses are trustworthy professionals (as discussed in Ch 5).

Writing an application letter

Generally, your **application letter** should specify the position (using the reference code from the employer), state your interest and briefly outline your eligibility and suitability for the job. It should be a short, business style letter. You must always address the criteria and provide any information required by the employer. For example, if you are advised to 'provide evidence of your recent experience in renal nursing in your application letter', you should do so. (See the 'Sample job application letter' (R7.4) in the 'Job application folio' (R7) on the CD Part 3—Reader resources.)

Preparing a curriculum vitae

A **curriculum vitae (CV)** or **resumé** is a very important document that provides a summary of your personal information, educational qualifications and employment history.

While CV formats can vary, they usually contain sections for demographic data, education/qualifications, employment history—with a very brief description of roles and responsibilities—personal interests and references. CVs are usually written in point form and it is essential that your CV is short (many places specify a maximum of 3 pages), and that the spelling and grammar are correct. Attach a certified copy of your visa to your CV. Ensure that your full name (as it appears on your visa), as well as any names by which you are known, is noted on your CV.

For assistance with preparing your CV, contact the study skills advisors at your educational institution, or a commercial CV preparation service (some specialise in CVs for nurses). (See the 'Sample curriculum vitae' (R7.5) in the 'Job application folio' (R7) on the CD Part 3—Reader resources.)

Providing references

You might be required to provide the contact details of personal and/or professional **referees**. If the number is not specified, provide at least two professional referees. List their names, positions and contact details in the **references** section of your CV. Often, an employer will telephone the referee. If a written reference is required, you must also provide the original letter.

It can sometimes be difficult for overseas nurses and international students to provide recent employment references, so you might need to provide a reference from a previous employer overseas. If so, this must be in writing, with a translation by a professional translator. Suitable local referees could include a teacher or clinical teacher or an employer (if you have been working in Australia or New Zealand).

Always ask permission before nominating someone as your referee. You should also provide a professional referee with the position description and a copy of your CV to assist them to address the relevant criteria when providing the reference for you.

Preparing for an interview

Before the interview

If you are successful in obtaining an **interview** for a job, it is important to be very well prepared for the interview. Research the facility, and be able to discuss its history, mission and the type of services it offers, and review the position description. Prepare a list of questions—about the organisation or the position—to ask at interview. Aim to have at least two questions, as this demonstrates your research and interest.

Know the location of the facility and organise your transport well in advance. If you are driving, ask about the parking available. Be certain you know where the interview will be conducted. It is best to obtain this in writing (to avoid any misunderstanding).

Presentation and conduct

Ensure that you arrive early for the interview. It is advisable to wear smart clothing and shoes and be very well groomed. Take a copy of the position description, your application and CV, your professional **portfolio** if you have been practising as a nurse (see Ch 5), and your list of questions.

You will be introduced to the **interviewers** at the start of the interview. Try to address them by name throughout the interview. It is polite and acceptable to use first names, unless a person is introduced differently. For example, if an interviewer is introduced as Tom Smith, you can call him 'Tom'; if an interviewer is introduced as Professor Baker, call her 'Professor' or 'Professor Baker'.

Interview formats

There are various interview formats, including group interviews and individual interviews, and sometimes a written test (e.g. drug calculations) is conducted at the interview.

During a group interview, you will be asked to work on a task as part of a small group. It is important to communicate clearly and effectively, as the interviewers will be observing your communication and team member skills, along with your knowledge. It is possible that individual interviews will be conducted as well as the group interview.

Individual interviews will usually be conducted by at least two interviewers. Sometimes, a panel of interviewers (of three or more) will interview **applicants**. Usually, the interviewers ask a series of questions and the applicant responds to the questions.

Interview questions

It is good to anticipate the questions you will be asked during an interview, so you can prepare your responses. Table 14.1 outlines some possible categories for interview questions. (See the 'Sample interview questions' (R7.6) in the 'Job application folio' (R7) on the CD Part 3—Reader resources.)

TABLE 14.1 Interview question categories

General interests
Qualifications and evidence of meeting mandatory criteria (e.g. registration as a nurse)
Employment history
Interest in position
Evidence of competence and specific experience, abilities and skills related to position description (may include case study or scenario questions, drug calculation competency test and other activities)
Evidence of knowledge of professional issues
Clarification of terms and conditions of employment
Opportunity for questions
Availability

After the interview

If your application and interview are successful, and the prospective employer is satisfied with the reference checks, you will normally be telephoned and offered the position. After you accept the offer, you will receive written confirmation of your appointment and at some stage will sign a contract with the employer.

It is possible that you will also be asked to consent to certain security procedures, such as a **police check**. This is often a condition of employment, and you will be asked to complete a special form, detailing personal information and advising if you have a police record. The form is submitted to the relevant police department and the records are checked to determine if you have a police record (for any criminal activity). The police department then notifies the employer of the outcome of the check. This is not related to being an international applicant, as all employees in some organisations are subject to the same condition.

If you are not successful in obtaining the position, it is acceptable to ask for feedback about your application. Try to address constructive feedback, particularly about your interview preparation or conduct, in future job applications.

CHAPTER HIGHLIGHTS

- Check relevant sources for job advertisements.
- Be aware of the initial position requirements and conditions, particularly that the organisation is a legitimate employer offering award wages and conditions.
- Before applying for a position, carefully consider the information in the position description and research the employer. Then check that your skills, experience, interests and aspirations match the position and the organisation.
- Applications usually require a letter and a CV to determine suitability for interview. Ensure that your written application is of a professional standard.
- Provide suitable references or nominate appropriate people as your referees. Always seek permission before nominating a referee.
- If you are offered an interview, prepare well, present yourself professionally and ask questions to demonstrate your understanding and interest.
- Obtain feedback about your application to assist with your professional development.

Self-test questions

Plain numbered questions are for all readers; 'a' questions are for readers in Australia; 'b' questions are for readers in New Zealand.

1. Find an advertisement for a nursing job in one of the common sources for nursing job advertisements in your area.

2a. Review the information about award wages and conditions for nurses on the Australian Nursing Federation (ANF) website: www.anf.org.au

2b. Review the information about award wages and conditions for nurses on the New Zealand Nurses Organisation (NZNO) website: www.nzno.org.nz

3. After reviewing the 'Sample curriculum vitae' (R7.5) in the 'Job application folio' (R7) on the CD Part 3—Reader resources, prepare your CV.

4a. Review the information about portfolios on the following websites:

Australian Nursing and Midwifery Council:
www.anmc.org.au/docs/Research%20and%20Policy/Continuing%20Competencies/National%20Continuing%20Competence%20Framework%20Draft%20v2%203.pdf

Australian Nursing Federation:
www.onwebfast.com/anf/pd_record_demo.htm

Nurses and Midwives Board of Western Australia:
www.nmbwa.org.au/1/1119/50/professional_co.pm

If you have been a registered nurse in the past, develop a professional portfolio.

4b. Review the information about portfolios on the following websites:

College of Nurses Aotearoa:
www.nurse.org.nz/guidelines/gl_portfolio.htm

New Zealand Nurses Organisation:
www.nzno.org.nz/Site/Resources/Portfolios.aspx

If you have been a registered nurse in the past, develop a professional portfolio.

5. Review the key terms and any other new vocabulary, terms and abbreviations from this chapter, and then update your 'Language list' (R2) on the CD Part 3—Reader resources.
6. Answer the 'Learning objectives' at the start of this chapter as if they were examination questions.

Recommended reading

Queensland University of Technology 2005 QUT student nurses get that job. Online. Available www.careers.qut.edu.au/job/applications/booklets/Nursing2005.pdf 30 Dec 2007

PART 7

Learning activities for use with CD

This section contains resources to assist your learning when you are using the CD. The activities and self-test questions are for use with the CD Part 1—Audio, 'Nursing conversations' (A4–A14) and 'Nursing handovers' (A15–A16).

You will need the following:

- the CD
- transcripts for A4–A16 (from the CD Part 2—Transcripts (T4–T16))
- pens: blue or black pen, red pen and green pen
- paper or a workbook, and
- the 'Nursing handover worksheets' (R12) for A15–A16 (from the CD Part 3—Reader resources).

Important note

Complete Part 1 of the 'Healthcare abbreviations self-directed learning package' (R11) ***before*** starting these activities. Listen to each track on the CD ***before*** you read these self-test questions. Then complete the relevant activities and self-test questions before listening to the following track. It is suggested that you use different coloured pens for each part of the activity (blue or black for first level—listening; red for second level—repeat listening; green for third level—reading transcript). This will allow you to self-assess your listening skills and, when you attempt these activities in the future, you will be able to monitor your progress.

Nursing conversations

Introduction

- Listen to A4.
- After the track has finished, make brief notes, outlining what you have heard.

Answer the following questions using a blue or black pen:

a. What is the patient's name?
b. What is the nurse's name?
c. What is the patient's preferred name?
d. During which shift does this conversation take place?

- Listen to A4 again.
- Using a red pen, correct your answers if necessary.
- Read the transcript for A4 (from the CD Part 2 (T4)).
- Using a green pen, correct your answers if necessary.

Social conversation

- Listen to A5.
- After the track has finished, make brief notes, outlining what you have heard.

Answer the following questions using a blue or black pen:

a. What are the main topics of the conversation?
b. What leisure activities does the patient like?
c. What leisure activities does the nurse like?
d. What season is it?

- Listen to A5 again.
- Using a red pen, correct your answers if necessary.
- Read the transcript for A5 (from the CD Part 2 (T5)).
- Using a green pen, correct your answers if necessary.

Admission interview

- Listen to A6.
- After the track has finished, make brief notes, outlining what you have heard.

Answer the following questions using a blue or black pen:

a. What is the patient's admission diagnosis?
b. List the patient's past health history.
c. What are the patient's current problems?
d. Describe the patient's allergy in detail.
e. What referral will the nurses make?

- Listen to A6 again.
- Using a red pen, correct your answers if necessary.
- Read the transcript for A6 (from the CD Part 2 (T6)).
- Using a green pen, correct your answers if necessary.

Performing clinical skills

- Listen to A7.
- After the track has finished, make brief notes, outlining what you have heard.

Answer the following questions using a blue or black pen:

a. What clinical skills does the nurse perform?
b. What does the nurse say to obtain consent before performing the clinical skills?
c. For *each* of the clinical skills, note the information the nurse gives the patient before she commences the skill.
d. What are the assessment findings for each clinical skill?
e. What action will the nurse take after she has completed the skills?

- Listen to A7 again.
- Using a red pen, correct your answers if necessary.
- Read the transcript for A7 (from the CD Part 2 (T7)).
- Using a green pen, correct your answers if necessary.

Mobilising and positioning a patient

- Listen to A8.
- After the track has finished, make brief notes, outlining what you have heard.

Answer the following questions using a blue or black pen:

a. Describe all of the positions the patient assumes throughout this conversation. List both the plain English and the medical terms for *each* position.
b. Where possible, provide rationales for each of the positions (i.e. why the patient assumes each position).

- Listen to A8 again.
- Using a red pen, correct your answers if necessary.
- Read the transcript for A8 (from the CD Part 2 (T8)).
- Using a green pen, correct your answers if necessary.

Reporting information

- Listen to A9.
- After the track has finished, make brief notes, outlining what you have heard.

Answer the following questions using a blue or black pen:

a. What does the nurse report?
b. To whom does the nurse report the information? What is the person's full name and position?
c. What is the nurse advised to do?
d. What information about the patient should be reported?
e. To whom should further reports be made?

- Listen to A9 again.
- Using a red pen, correct your answers if necessary.
- Read the transcript for A9 (from the CD Part 2 (T9)).
- Using a green pen, correct your answers if necessary.

Referral

- Listen to A10.
- After the track has finished, make brief notes, outlining what you have heard.

Answer the following questions using a blue or black pen:

a. To whom does the nurse make a referral? What is the person's name, profession and position?
b. What is the patient's name?
c. What is the reason for the referral?
d. When will the patient be reviewed (by the person who receives the referral)?

- Listen to A10 again.
- Using a red pen, correct your answers if necessary.
- Read the transcript for A10 (from the CD Part 2 (T10)).
- Using a green pen, correct your answers if necessary.

Telephone conversation

- Listen to A11.
- After the track has finished, make brief notes, outlining what you have heard.

Answer the following questions using a blue or black pen:

a. What is the nurse's name?
b. Who is the caller? What is the person's full name and position?
c. What is the purpose of the telephone call?
d. What specific information does the caller provide?
e. What action does the nurse plan to take after the call has finished?

- Listen to A11 again.
- Using a red pen, correct your answers if necessary.
- Read the transcript for A11 (from the CD Part 2 (T11)).
- Using a green pen, correct your answers if necessary.

Patient education

- Listen to A12.
- After the track has finished, make brief notes, outlining what you have heard.

Answer the following questions using a blue or black pen:

a. What is the nurse teaching the patient?
b. What concerns does the patient have?
c. List in detail how the nurse addresses the patient's concerns.
d. During which shift does this conversation take place?

- Listen to A12 again.
- Using a green pen, correct your answers if necessary.
- Read the transcript for A12 (from the CD Part 2 (T12)).
- Using a green pen, correct your answers if necessary.

Discharge

- Listen to A13.
- After the track has finished, make brief notes, outlining what you have heard.

Answer the following questions using a blue or black pen:

a. When is the patient being discharged?
b. What is the discharge destination (where is the patient going)?
c. Who will collect the patient?
d. What are the discharge transport arrangements?
e. What specific discharge education is provided to the patient?
f. What arrangements have been made for follow-up appointments?

- Listen to A13 again.
- Using a red pen, correct your answers if necessary.
- Read the transcript for A13 (from the CD Part 2 (T13)).
- Using a green pen, correct your answers if necessary.

Concluding conversation

- Listen to A14.
- After the track has finished, make brief notes, outlining what you have heard.

Answer the following questions using a blue or black pen:

a. What is the nurse's name?
b. What does the patient ask the nurse to do before she leaves?
c. During which shift does this conversation take place?

- Listen to A14 again.
- Using a red pen, correct your answers if necessary.

- Read the transcript for A14 (from the CD Part 2 (T14)).
- Using a green pen, correct your answers if necessary.

Nursing handovers

Morning shift

- Listen to A15 and take notes *while* you are listening.
- Answer the following questions using a blue or black pen. You can refer to your own handover notes.
- Answer Questions a–j on the 'Morning shift' worksheet in the 'Nursing handover worksheets' (R12) (see the CD Part 3—Reader resources).

For each patient list their:

a. bed number
b. name
c. age
d. day of stay
e. admission diagnosis
f. past health history
g. mobility
h. level of independence with activities of daily living
i. current care/management
j. referrals or reviews
k. Which patients are in the preoperative phase?
l. Why is the physiotherapist coming to the ward this afternoon?
m. Who reviewed the patient in bed 3 this morning, and what treatment was prescribed?
n. Which patients require referral to or review by another health professional, and why?

- Listen to A15 again.
- Using a red pen, correct your answers if necessary.
- Read the transcript for A15 (from the CD Part 2 (T15)).
- Using a green pen, correct your answers if necessary.

Advanced learning activities

- *Listening and speaking*: After you have completed this activity, practise handing over the information to a fellow student or colleague. Compare your handover notes with each other, and with the transcript. Discuss the reasons for any differences or inaccuracies.
- *Documentation*: Rewrite the transcript for each patient, as if it was a set of nursing notes. Use the information listed in Tables 11.2 and 11.4 of the text to assist you. Check your work using the 'Nursing documentation checklist' (R6.8) in the 'Clinical placement folio' (R6) on the CD Part 3—Reader resources.
- *Clinical nursing care*: Formulate a comprehensive nursing care plan for each patient. Use the 'Preparation for patient care document' (R6.6) in the 'Clinical

placement folio' (R6) on the CD Part 3—Reader resources. Ensure that you have addressed the information listed in Tables 13.2 and 13.3 of the text.

Afternoon shift

- Listen to A16 and take notes *while* you are listening.
- Answer the following questions using a blue or black pen. You can refer to your own handover notes.
- Answer Questions a–j on the 'Afternoon shift' worksheet in the 'Nursing handover worksheets' (R12) (see the CD Part 3—Reader resources).

For each patient list their:

a. bed number
b. name
c. age
d. day of stay
e. admission diagnosis
f. past health history
g. mobility
h. level of independence with activities of daily living
i. current care/management
j. referrals or reviews
k. Which patients have intravenous therapy in situ?
l. Which patients are in the postoperative phase?
m. What problem did the patient in bed 3 experience this afternoon, and what ongoing management is required?
n. Which patients require referral to or review by another health professional, and why?

- Listen to A16 again.
- Using a red pen, correct your answers if necessary.
- Read the transcript for A16 (from the CD Part 2 (T16)).
- Using a green pen, correct your answers if necessary.

Advanced learning activities

- *Listening and speaking*: After you have completed this activity, practise handing over the information to a fellow student or colleague. Compare your handover notes with each other, and with the transcript. Discuss the reasons for any differences or inaccuracies.
- *Documentation*: Rewrite the transcript for each patient, as if it was a set of nursing notes. Use the information listed in Tables 11.2 and 11.4 of the text to assist you. Check your work using the 'Nursing documentation checklist' (R6.8) in the 'Clinical placement folio' (R6) on the CD Part 3—Reader resources.
- *Clinical nursing care*: Formulate a comprehensive nursing care plan for each patient. Use the 'Preparation for patient care document' (R6.6) in the 'Clinical placement folio' (R6) on the CD Part 3—Reader resources. Ensure that you have addressed the information listed in Tables 13.2 and 13.3 of the text.

Index

Page numbers followed by 'b' denote boxes, 'f' denote figures and 't' denote tables.